Mullaicharam Bhupathyraaj

Quality Control for Pharmaceutical and Cosmetic Preparations

Mullaicharam Bhupathyraaj

Quality Control for Pharmaceutical and Cosmetic Preparations

Dosage form and Quality Control

Noor Publishing

Imprint

Any brand names and product names mentioned in this book are subject to trademark, brand or patent protection and are trademarks or registered trademarks of their respective holders. The use of brand names, product names, common names, trade names, product descriptions etc. even without a particular marking in this work is in no way to be construed to mean that such names may be regarded as unrestricted in respect of trademark and brand protection legislation and could thus be used by anyone.

Cover image: www.ingimage.com

Publisher:
Noor Publishing
is a trademark of
Dodo Books Indian Ocean Ltd. and OmniScriptum S.R.L publishing group

120 High Road, East Finchley, London, N2 9ED, United Kingdom
Str. Armeneasca 28/1, office 1, Chisinau MD-2012, Republic of Moldova, Europe
Printed at: see last page
ISBN: 978-620-5-63462-2

S.No.	Topic
1.	**CHAPTER-1** Introduction to quality control of pharmaceuticals & concept of Laboratory Practice.
2.	**CHAPTER-2** Concepts related to quality control of pharmaceutical products. Evaluation of Quality of drug products.
3.	**CHAPTER-3** Quality Standards and Compendial Requirements for tablets. Quality control tests for tablets- hardness, friability, thickness, c
4.	**CHAPTER-4** Quality Standards and Compendial Requirements for capsules.
5.	**CHAPTER-5** Evaluate the oral liquid preparations and their packaging materi
6.	**CHAPTER-6** Evaluation of cosmetic products - Hair Cosmetics-Shampoo
7.	**CHAPTER-7** Evaluation of cosmetic products - Skin Cosmetics- Lipstick
8.	**CHAPTER-8** Quality control of vaccines
9.	**CHAPTER-9** Good manufacturing practice
10.	**CHAPTER-10** Good Compounding Practices

CHAPTER 1

troduction to Quality Control of Pharmaceuticals & Concept of Good Laboratory Practice.

ing objectives:

ompletion of this unit, students should be able to

Learn important concepts related to quality control of pharmaceutical products.

Understand the impact of low-quality medicines on health in general.

Explain determinants of medicine quality and their method of assessment and evaluation.

iew of Lecture 1

Introduction

Difference between QA and QC

QC of pharmaceutical products

Impact of low quality medicines on health

Determinants of medicine quality

Introduction:

Glossary of commonly used terms in Pharmaceutical industry

Active Pharmaceutical Ingredient (API)

- Any substance or mixture of substances intended to be used in the manufacture of a pharmaceutical dosage form and that, when so used, becomes an active ingredient of that pharmaceutical dosage form.
- Such substances are intended to furnish pharmacological activity or other direct effect in the diagnosis, cure, mitigation, treatment, or prevention of disease or to affect the structure and function of the body.

Finished Product

- A finished dosage form that has undergone all stages of manufacture, including packaging in its final container and labelling.

Intermediate Product

- Partly processed product that must undergo further manufacturing steps before it becomes a bulk product.

Pharmaceutical Product

- Any material or product intended for human or veterinary use presented in its finished dosage form or as a starting material for use in such a dosage form, that is subject to control by pharmaceutical legislation in the exporting state and/or the importing state.

In-process Control

- Checks performed during production in order to monitor and, if necessary, to adjust the process to ensure that the product conforms to its specifications.

- The control of the environment or equipment may also be regarded as a part of in process control.

Manufacture

- All operations of purchase of materials and products, production, quality control, release, storage and distribution of pharmaceutical products, and the related controls

Packaging Material

- Any material, including printed material, employed in the packaging of a pharmaceutical, but excluding any outer packaging used for transportation or shipment. Packaging materials are referred to as primary or secondary according to whether or not they are intended to be in direct contact with the product.

Production

- All operations involved in the preparation of a pharmaceutical product, from receipt of materials, through processing, packaging and repackaging, labelling and relabeling, to completion of the finished product.

In-process Control

- Checks performed during production in order to monitor and, if necessary, to adjust the process to ensure that the product conforms to its specifications.
- The control of the environment or equipment may also be regarded as a part of in process control.

Manufacture

- All operations of purchase of materials and products, production, quality control, release, storage and distribution of pharmaceutical products, and the related controls

Packaging Material

- Any material, including printed material, employed in the packaging of a pharmaceutical, but excluding any outer packaging used for transportation or shipment. Packaging materials are referred to as primary or secondary according to whether or not they are intended to be in direct contact with the product.

Production

- All operations involved in the preparation of a pharmaceutical product, from receipt of materials, through processing, packaging and repackaging, labelling and relabeling, to completion of the finished product.

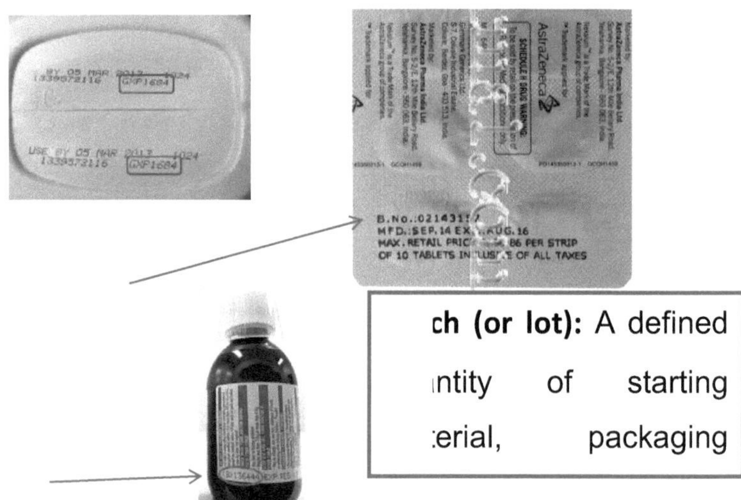

Large-volume parenterals (LVP): Sterile solutions intended for parenteral application with a volume of 100 ml or more in one container of the finished dosage form.

Quarantine: The status of starting or packaging materials, intermediates, or bulk or finished products isolated physically or by other effective means while a decision is awaited on their release, rejection or reprocessing.

- **Specification:** A list of detailed requirements with which the products or materials used or obtained during manufacture have to conform. They serve as a basis for quality evaluation.

- **Standard Operating Procedure (SOP):** An authorized written procedure giving instructions for performing operations not necessarily specific to a given product or material (e.g. equipment operation, maintenance and cleaning; cleaning of premises etc).

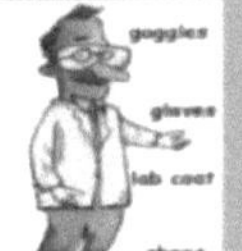

Calibration

To ensure that instruments producing accurate results.

Validation

Documented evidence that a process, equipment, method or system produce consistent result (uniform batch produced)

Key Definitions

Pharmaceutical Quality Assurance

Pharmaceutical quality assurance may be defined as the sum of all activities and responsibilities required to ensure that the medicine that reaches the patient is safe, effective, and acceptable to the patient.

Pharmaceutical Quality Control

As defined by WHO, quality control is the part of the firm's process concerned with medicine sampling, specifications, testing, and the organization's release procedures that ensure that the necessary tests are carried out and that the materials are not released for use, nor products released for sale or supply, until their quality has been judged satisfactory.

Quality System, Quality Assurance, and Quality Control Relationships

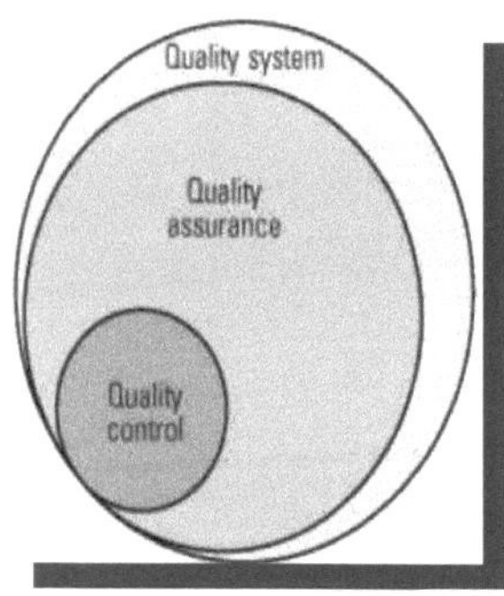

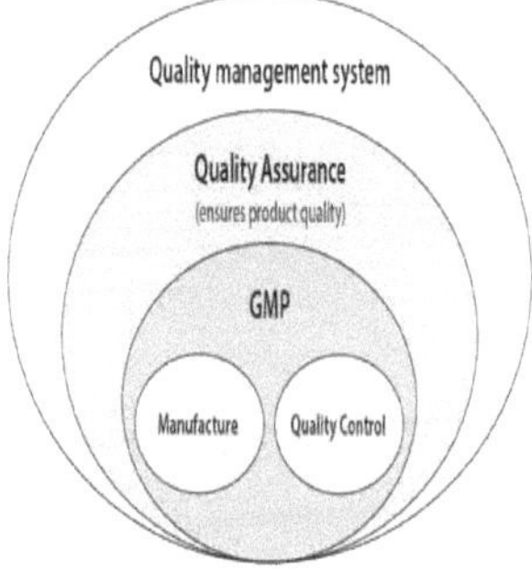

Quality Assurance (QA)

- ➡ QA is process oriented and focuses on defect prevention.
- ➡ Improves processes used to develop products (Proactive process)
- ➡ QA refers to the process used to create the deliverables, and can be performed by manager, client, or even a third-party reviewer.

- Quality assurance is a much wider concept: Covers all matters which individually or collectively influence the quality of a product.
- QA= GCPs + GMPs + GLPs
- Final testing of the product cannot ensure the quality, safety, efficacy of a product Therefore the concept of QC evolved
- The development of QC resulted in GMPs
- Examples; process checklists and improvement (methodology), selection of tools and education.

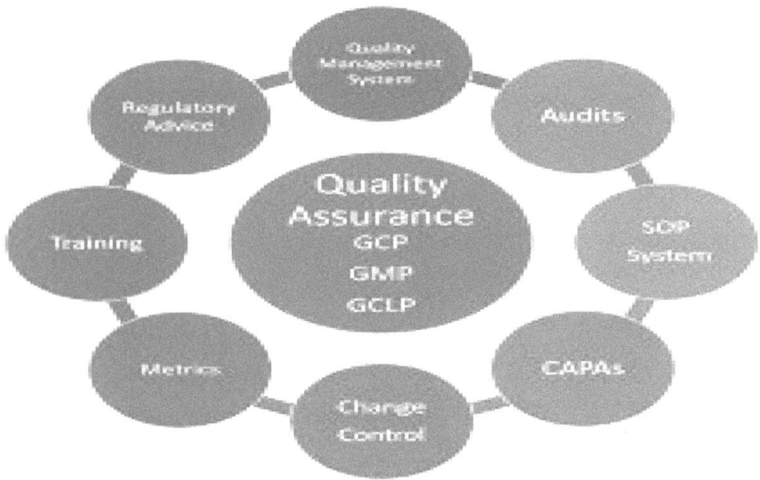

- QA activities are determined <u>before production work begins</u> and these activities are <u>performed while the product is being developed</u>.

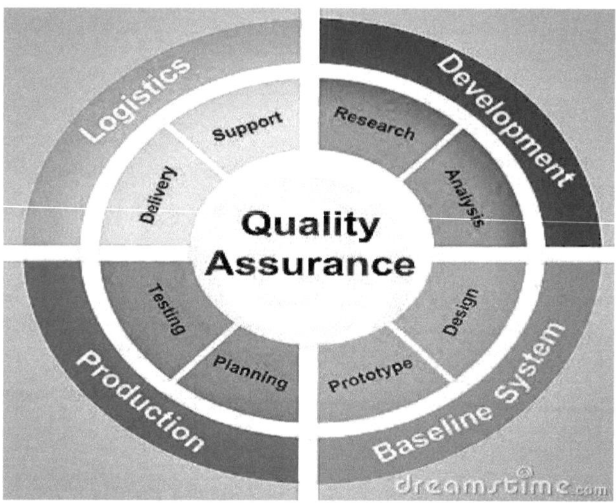

Quality control (QC)

➡ https://youtu.be/P8H0MR4PtWw

Quality control (QC)

- QC is *product* oriented and focuses on defect *identification*.
- QC is used to verify that deliverables are of acceptable quality and that they are complete and correct.
- Examples of QC activities include
- inspection,
- test design and
- test execution.
- QC activities are performed after the product is developed but before it is released
- https://www.youtube.com/watch?v=yhZ6Mg3FQSI

COMPONENTS OF QC

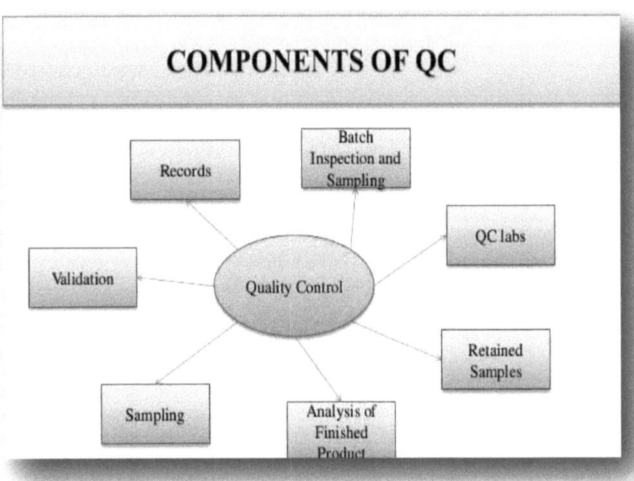

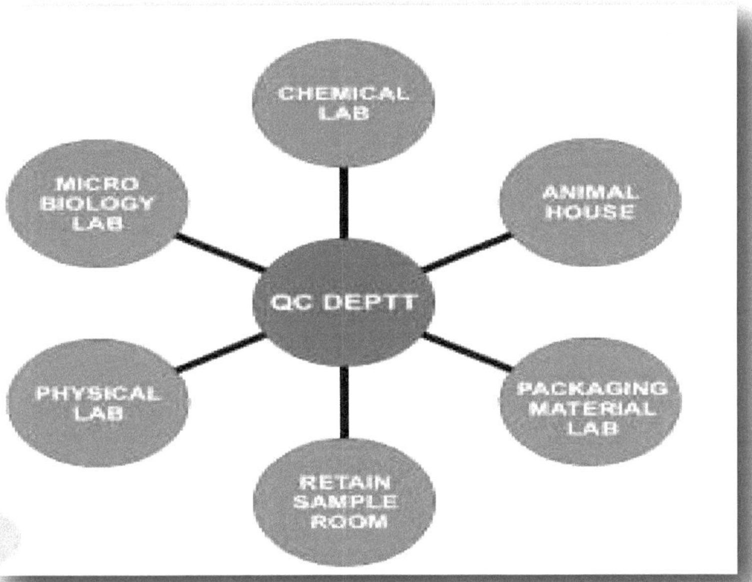

Responsibilities of Quality Control personnel

- To follow the laid down safety precautions while working in the laboratory.
- Maintenance or upkeep of Laboratory working area.
- Ensure compliance with current Good Laboratory Practices and current Good Manufacturing Practices.
- Sampling of Purified / Potable Water and its analysis.
- Analysis of Raw Materials (API / Excipients), Analysis of finished Product, Packing Material, In process samples and Stability Sample. Qualification of Laboratory Instruments and Equipment's.
- Daily Calibration and Monthly Calibration of Analytical Balances and other Instruments.
- Preparation of Calibration Schedules and ensure for proper execution.
- Preparation of Specification of Raw, Packing, In process & Finished products.
- Preparation of Standard Test Procedure for Raw, Packing, In process & Finished products.
- Reporting of Incidence, Out of Specification and Out of Trend results observed during analysis.
- Preparation of Certificate of Analysis (COA) .
- Preparation of Stability summary after analysis.
- Status labeling of Quality control instruments, Chemicals & Glassware.
- Disposal of balance samples after completion of analysis and its documentation.

	Quality Assurance	**Quality control**
Definition	QA is a set of activities for <u>ensuring quality in the processes</u> by which products are developed	Set of activities for <u>ensuring quality in products</u>. The activities focus on <u>identifying defects</u> in the actual products produced.
Focus on	QA aims to <u>prevent defects</u> with a <u>focus on the process</u> used to make the product. It is a **proactive quality** process.	QC aims to <u>identify (and correct) defects in the finished product</u>. Quality control, therefore, is a **reactive process.**
Goal	The goal of QA is to improve development and test processes so that defects do not arise when the product is being developed.	The goal of QC is to identify defects after a product is developed and before it's released.
How	Establish a good quality management system and the assessment of its adequacy. Periodic conformance audits of the operations of the system.	Finding & eliminating sources of quality problems through tools & equipment so that customer's requirements are continually met.
What	Prevention of quality problems through planned and systematic activities including documentation.	The activities or techniques used to achieve and maintain the product quality, process and service.
Responsibility	Everyone on the team involved in developing the product is responsible for quality assurance.	Quality control is usually the responsibility of a specific team that tests the product for defects.
As a tool	QA is a managerial tool	QC is a corrective tool

Understand impact of low quality medicines on health in general

Impact of Low-Quality Medicines

During

- Manufacturing process
- Packaging
- Transportation
- Storage condition

Lack of therapeutic effect: Prolonged illness, Death, Toxic and adverse reaction, Waste of limited Financial resources, Loss of credibility

Determinants of Medicine Quality

- Identity: Active ingredient (The correct active ingredient is present)
- Purity: Not contaminated with potentially harmful

substances

- Potency: Usually 90–110% of the labeled amount
- Uniformity: Consistency of color, shape, size
- Bioavailability: Interchangeable products
- Stability: Ensuring medicine activity for stated period

- Identity, purity, potency, uniformity are defined in pharmacopoeias and stated in certificate of analysis (COA)

Certificate of analysis

A certificate of analysis is prepared for each batch of a substance or product and usually contains the following information:
   (a) the registration number of the sample;
   (b) date of receipt;
   (c) the name and address of the laboratory testing the sample;
   (d) the name and address of the originator of the request for analysis;
   (e) the name, description and batch number of the sample where appropriate;
   (f) the name and address of the original manufacturer and, if applicable, those of the repacked and/or trader;
   (g) the reference to the specification used for testing the sample;
   (h) the results of all tests performed (mean and standard deviation, if applicable) with the prescribed limits;
   (i) a conclusion as to whether or not the sample was found to be within the limits of the specification;
   (j) expiry date or retest date if applicable;
   (k) date on which the test(s) was (were) completed; and
   (l) The signature of the head of laboratory or other authorized person.

**How Is Quality
Assessed?**

- **INSPECTION** of products on arrival

    - Visual inspection

    - Product specification review (including expiration dates)

- **LABORATORY TESTING** for compliance with pharmacopoeial standards

    - International Pharmacopoeia

    - European Pharmacopoeia

    - U. S. Pharmacopeia

    - British Pharmacopoeia

    - National Pharmacopoeia

- **BIOAVAILABILITY DATA**

Raw Materials (API, inert)

- All Raw Materials are tested on site before use

    - Incoming identity

    - Full release testing

    - (receiving area, stored, color coded, yellow, red, green)

- Includes Excipients, Capsules, API

- Various techniques

    - Spectroscopic techniques

    - Assay (HPLC and Titration)

    - Physical Tests (Particle size, heavy metal content, residue on ignition,
      pH, foreign matter, microbial limit)

> **All packaging components tested if in contact with drug product**
> > Bottles
> > Blister pack components
> > Cotton wool, Desiccants
> > **Range of techniques**
> > Appearance
> > Spectroscopy
> > Loss on Drying

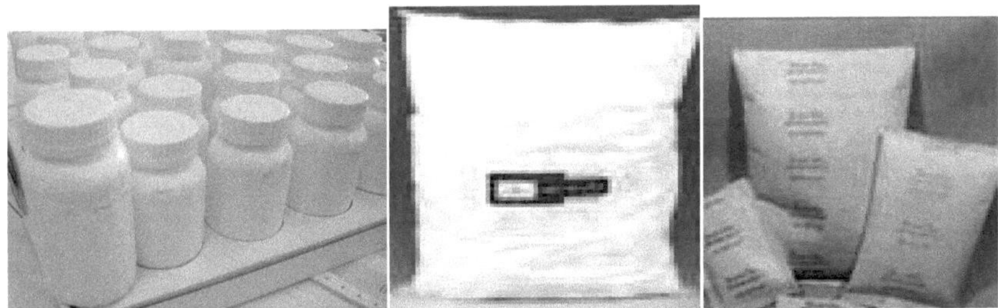

Finished Product (Release)

- **Release into Clinic**
- **Mainly 2 techniques**
  - HPLC
  - Dissolution
- **Several tests**
  - Assay
  - Content Uniformity
  - Dissolution

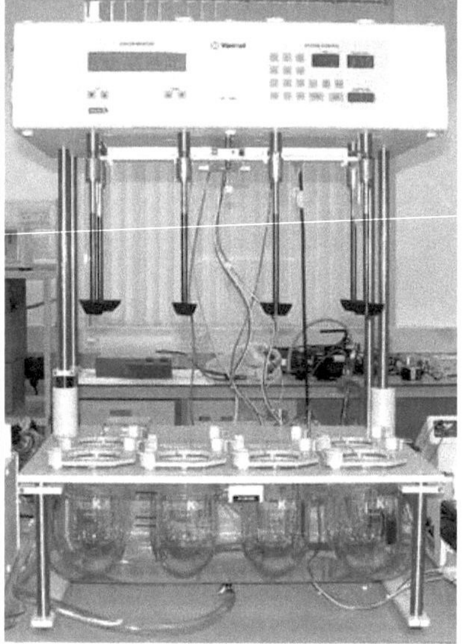

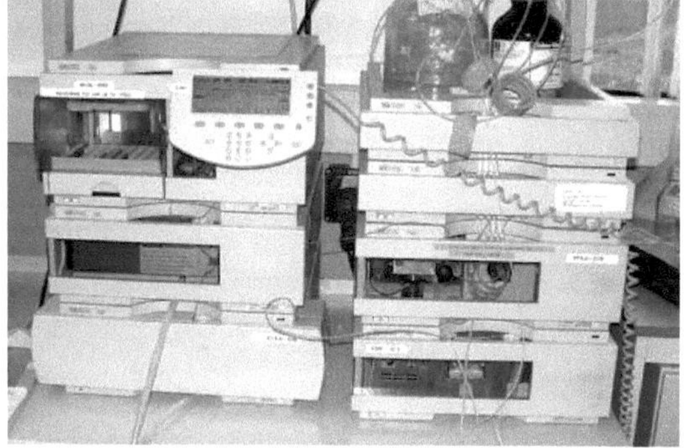

Retains

- Sample of everything tested retained
  - Enough for full testing in duplicate
  - At label conditions

➡ Retain time determined by regulatory guidelines

- ➡ Raw materials 12 Years

- ➡ Finished products 10 Years

➡ All unsealed finished products inspected annually

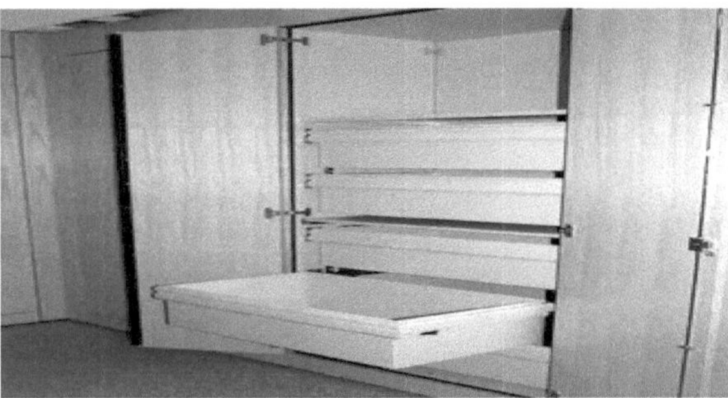

Retained samples:

Samples should be retained as required by the legislation or by the originator of the request for analysis.

There should be a sufficient

amount of retained sample to allow at least two re-analyses.

The retained sample should be kept in its final pack.

Cleaning Verification

- ➡ The company should describe the policy and approach to cleaning verification.

    Cleaning verification is

- ➡ where the effectiveness of the validated cleaning procedure is routinely verified. ➡ The approach may include swab or rinse samples.

- ➡ The results obtained from testing on a routine basis should be reviewed and subjected to statistical trending.

- ➡ Tested using HPLC

    - ➡ Swab concentration must be lower than std

- ➡ All surfaces must be validated

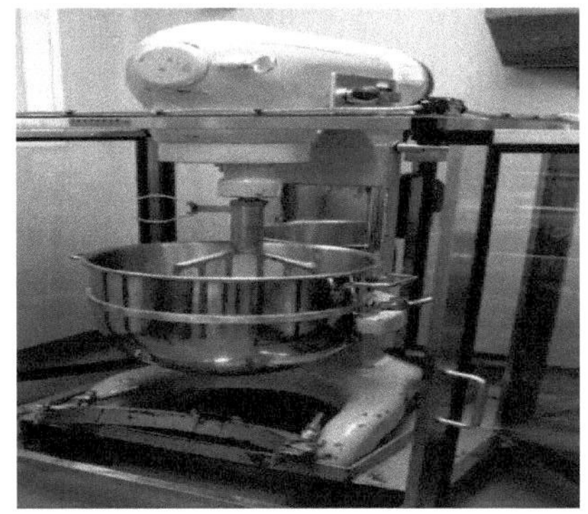

Learning outcomes

1. Gain knowledge related to QA, QC processes in the pharmaceutical industries.

2. Explain determinants of medicine quality and

3. Explain their method of assessment and evaluation.

- **Evaluation of quality of a drug product**

Overview

- Evaluation of quality of a drug product
- Quality assurance data:

Sources of specifications

Types of specifications

Finished product specifications

Release specifications

Stability testing studies

- Generally acceptable specifications for drug products
- Enlist the specifications of pharmaceutical products
- Concept of Good Laboratory Practice

Who Ensures Medicine Quality?

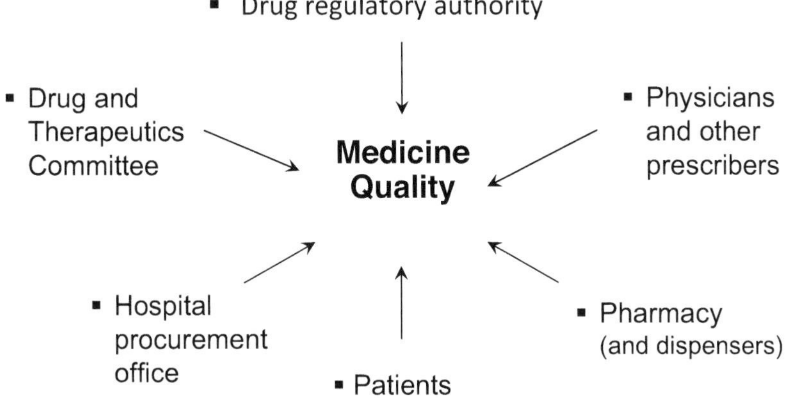

EVALUATION OF QUALITY OF A DRUG PRODUCT

Stages of new drug development

Research concept & discovery of lead compound

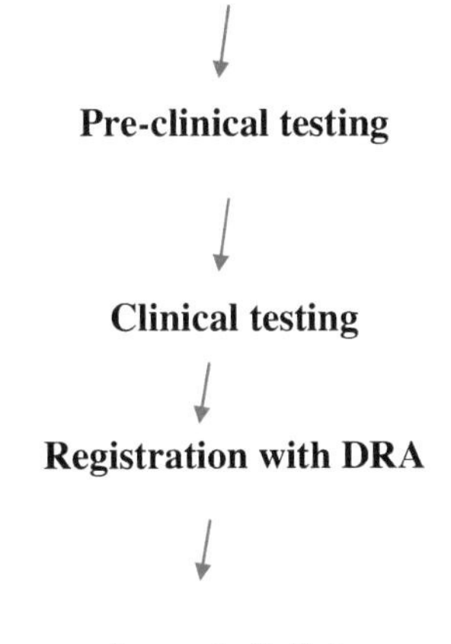

Pharmacy and chemical development works at each research phase

I Research concept and discovery of active lead compound

(Involves 8,000-10,000 potential candidate substances)

- Focuses mainly on ***extraction/synthesis*** of active substances at laboratory scale

II Preclinical testing

Selection of product candidate (basic pharmacology/biochemical screening) (20-30 substances reach this stage)

2.   Biological testing (pharmacological/toxicological studies)- (5-10 substances reach this stage)-

3. Clinical trials (phase I-II)-(Approximately 4-5 substances remain)

4. Registration with health authorities- (1 substance remain)

5. Launch and sales

ALTY ASSURANCE DATA

<u>**Specifications**</u>

Describe in detail the requirements with which products or materials used or obtained during manufacturing have to conform. *They serve as yard sticks for quality evaluation*

<u>**Sources of specifications**</u>

- Pharmacopeial
- In-house

<u>**Types of specifications**</u>

- Raw material specifications
- Container closure specifications
- Finished product specifications

<u>**Finished product specifications**</u>

- Release specifications
- Stability indicating specifications

<u>**Release specifications**</u>

The combinations of physical, chemical, biological and microbiological test requirements that determine whether a <u>drug product</u> is suitable for release at the time of manufacture.

<u>**Stability indicating specifications**</u>

The combination of physical, chemical, biological and microbiological test requirements that the active ingredients or a drug product must meet during its shelf life

Accelerated Stability testing (AST/ASA):

- **Definition:** Studies designed to increase the rate of chemical degradation and physical change of an API by using exaggerated storage conditions.
- **Purpose**: to provide evidence of how the quality of an API varies with time under the influence of temp, humidity and light (environmental factors).
- **Result of testing**: shelf life can be established and storage conditions are recommended.

Finished Pharmaceutical product (FPP): A product that has undergone all stages of production, including packaging in its final container and labeling. It may contain one or more APIs.

- <u>Long term and short term </u>(accelerated) storage conditions for **stability testing**:

➡ **For general products**

Study	Storage conditions	Minimum time period
Long term	$30\ ^{0}C\pm2$ / 65%±5 RH	12 months (up to 3 yrs)
Accelerated	$40\ ^{0}C\pm2$ / 75%±5 RH	6 months (data at 0, 3 and 6 months)

APIs intended for storage in a Refrigerator

Study	Storage conditions	Minimum time period
Long term	$5\ ^{0}C\pm3$	12 months (up to 3 yrs)
Accelerated	$30\ ^{0}C\pm2$ / 65%±5 RH	6 months (data at 0, 3 and 6 months)

Additional labeling statements for use where the result of stability testing demonstrates limiting factors

Limiting factors	:ional labeling statements, where

	relevant
FPPs that can not tolerate **refrigeration**	"Do not refrigerate or freeze"
FPPs that can not tolerate **freezing**	"Do not freeze"
Light sensitive FPPs	"Protect from light"
FPPs that can not tolerate excessive **heat**, eg. suppositories	"Store and transport not above 30^{0} C"
Hygroscopic FPPs	" Store in dry conditions"

EXAMPLES OF SPECIFICATIONS

Active pharmaceutical ingredients (API)

- Identity
- Purity
- Content
- Physico chemical properties such as solubility, melting points, particle size, etc.
- P^{H}

Finished product specifications

General

- Organoleptic properties (appearance, color, odor, shape)
- Identification
- Purity

- P^H
- Moisture content
- Abnormal toxicity

<u>Specific</u>

Tablet – dissolution/disintegration, weight variation, uniformity of content, friability/hardness, water content etc

Capsules – dissolution/disintegration, weight variation, brittleness (hard gelatin) water content, level of microbial contamination etc

For soft gelatin capsules, the fill medium should be examined for leakage, precipitate, cloudiness and pH

Generally acceptable specifications for drug products

Emulsions: - Appearance (such as phase separation), color, odor, pH, viscosity and strength.

➡ Storage on the side or inverted position.

➡ Heating and cooling cycle (4 and 45^0C).

Oral solutions and suspensions: Appearance (pH and cloudiness), strength, pH, color, odor, redispersibility, dissolution (suspension), clarity (solution)

➡ Storage on side or inverted position

➡ Assay

Oral powders: Reconstituted prior to administration. Examine for

➡ **Appearance**

➡ **strength**

➡ **Color, odor and moisture**

➡ **Water content and reconstitution time**

- Reconstituted product should be examined for **appearance, pH, dispersibility and strength throughout recommended storage period**.

Metered dose inhalation (MDIs) Aerosols:
- Strength
- Delivered dose per actuation
- No of metered doses
- Color
- Clarity (solutions)
- Particle size distribution (suspension)
- Pressure
- Valve corrosion
- Spray pattern

Topical and ophthalmic preparations

  (ointments, creams, lotions, pastes, gel and solutions)
- Appearance, clarity, color, homogeneity, odor, pH, resuspendability (lotions), consistency, <u>particle size</u> distribution, strength and <u>weight loss (plastic containers)</u>
- The <u>ophthalmic preparation needs tests for sterility</u>.
- Ointments, creams and pastes in <u>container **larger than 3.5 g**</u> should be assayed by **sampling at surface, middle and bottom** of container.

Small volume parenterals (SVP):
- Strength, appearance, color, particulate matter
- pH
- <u>Sterility and pyrogenicity</u>
- Stability studies on powder products
- Container closure integrity testing

➥ Preservative testing if present

Suppositories:

- Strength
- Softening range
- Appearance and dissolution at 37 ^{0}C
- Effect of ageing
- <u>Concept of Good Laboratory Practice</u>
- The history of GLP.
- The formal, regulatory, concept of "Good Laboratory Practice" (GLP) originated in the USA in the 1970s because of concerns about the validity of non-clinical safety data submitted to the Food and Drug Administration (FDA) in the context of New Drug Applications (NDA).
- The inspection of studies and test facilities revealed instances of inadequate planning and incompetent execution of studies, insufficient documentation of methods and results, and even cases of fraud.
- For example, replacing animals which had died during a study with new ones (which had not been treated appropriately with the test compound) without documenting this fact; taking hematology data for control animals from control groups not connected with the study; deleting gross necropsy observations because the histopathologist received no specimens of these lesions; and retrospectively changing raw data in order to "fit the result tables" in the final report.
- What is GLP?
- Good Laboratory Practice is defined in the OECD Principles as "a quality system concerned with the organizational process and the conditions under which non-clinical health and environmental safety studies are planned, performed, monitored, recorded, archived and reported."

- The purpose of the Principles of Good Laboratory Practice is to promote the development of quality test data and provide a tool to ensure a sound approach to the management of
- laboratory studies, including
- conduct,
- reporting and
- archiving.
- As far as pharmaceutical development is concerned, the GLP Principles, in their regulatory sense, apply only to studies which:
- • **are non-clinical**, i.e. mostly studies on animals or in vitro, including the analytical aspects of such studies;
- • **are designed to obtain data on the properties and/or the safety of items** with respect to human health and/or the environment;
- • **are intended to be submitted to a national registration authority** with the purpose of registering or licensing the tested substance or any product derived from it.

Depending on national legal situations, the GLP requirements for non-clinical laboratory studies conducted to evaluate drug safety cover the following classes of studies:

- Single dose toxicity
- Repeated dose toxicity (sub-acute and chronic)
- Reproductive toxicity (fertility, embryo-fetal toxicity and teratogenicity, peri-/post-natal toxicity)
- Mutagenic potential
- Carcinogenic potential
- Toxicokinetics (pharmacokinetic studies which provide systemic exposure data for the above studies)
- Pharmacodynamic studies designed to test the potential for adverse effects (Safety pharmacology)

- Local tolerance studies, including photo toxicity, irritation and sensitization studies, or testing for suspected addictive and/or withdrawal effects of drugs.

 GLP Principles are independent of the site where studies are performed. They apply to studies planned and conducted in a manufacturer's laboratory, at a contract or subcontract facility, or in a university or public sector laboratory.

THE FUNDAMENTAL POINTS OF GLP

Whatever the industry targeted, GLP stresses the importance of the following main points:

1. **Resources**: Organization, personnel, facilities and equipment;

2. **Characterization**: Test items and test systems;

3. **Rules**: Protocols, standard operating procedures (SOPs);

4. **Results**: Raw data, final report and archives;

5. **Quality Assurance**: Independent monitoring of research processes

Learning outcomes

1.Gain knowledge related to Evaluation of quality of a drug product

2. Explain Quality assurance data:

Sources of specifications

Types of specifications

Finished product specifications

Release specifications

Stability testing studies

3.Enlist the Generally acceptable specifications for drug products

4.Understand concept of Good Laboratory Practice

CHAPTER 2

Quality control of pharmaceutical products

Quality control of pharmaceutical products

<u>Learning objectives</u>

Upon completion of this unit, student should be able to

1. Learn the relationships among Fitness for Use, Quality Attributes and Clinical Performance.
2. Understand the role of QA in Drug development.
3. Understand the role of QA in Drug Manufacturing
4. Enlist the Analytical techniques in pharmaceutical analysis
5. Identify the common sources of impurities in pharmaceutical products.

The Pharmaceutical Quality System (PQS)-Introduction

- A robust PQS is critical to assuring drug products are manufactured to meet the desired quality and performance attributes
- PQS is the key system evaluated during FDA inspection, and is also key in providing FDA confidence that appropriate (science and risk based) support information is used to make decisions (e.g., in submissions).

What is Quality of a pharmaceutical product?

- "It delivers the properties described on the label and is not contaminated" –Dr. Woodcock
- "fitness for intended use"[*]
- "freedom from defects"[*]
- "meeting or exceeding customer expectations"[*]
- "customer's definition of quality is the only one that matters"[*]

Customers are often not able to independently assess the quality of the drugs they use.

For a Drug Product, Typically the Patient Cannot "See" Quality!
Which product is sub-potent?

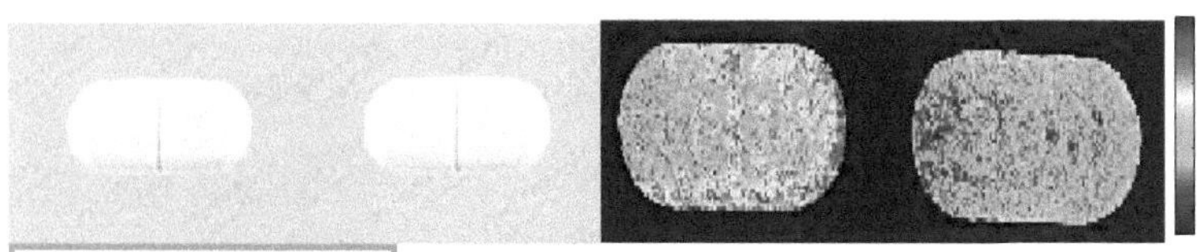

The Patient Expects Quality!!

Expectations for Quality

Patients and caregivers assume that their drugs

- Are safe, efficacious, and have the correct identity
- Deliver the same performance as described in the label
- Perform consistently over their shelf life
- Are made in a manner that ensures quality
- Will be available when needed

What really assures Quality?

- 1• QS Elements   / Framework - ICH Q10 (international Council for Harmonization of Technical Requirements for Pharmaceuticals
- 2• FDA Evaluation – Inspection & Review
- 3• Standards& Expectations – Regulations & CGMPs

Background: ICH Q10 - Pharmaceutical Quality SystemThe pharmaceutical quality system "assures that the desired product quality is routinely met, suitable process performance is achieved, the set of controls are appropriate, improvement opportunities are identified and evaluated, and the body of knowledge is continually expanded."

ICH Q10, Section 3.1.3 Commercial Manufacturing

ICH Q10 - Pharmaceutical Quality System

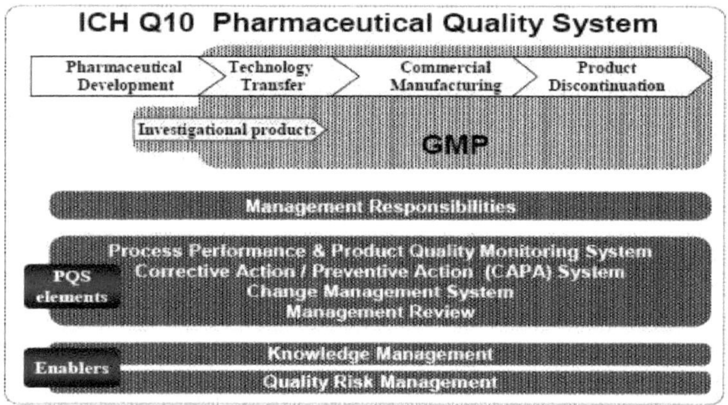

Four Pharmaceutical QS elements

1. Process performance and product quality monitoring system

2. Corrective action and preventive action (CAPA) system

3. Change management system

4. Management review of process performance and product quality

FDA Evaluation of PQS on Inspection

- **QS assessment is two phased:**
  - **Quality (Control) Unit has fulfilled responsibilities** – review & approve
  - **Assess Data collected to quality issues**
    - link **to other systems**
      - Facilities & Equipment
      - Materials
      - Production
      - Packaging & Labeling
      - Laboratory Controls

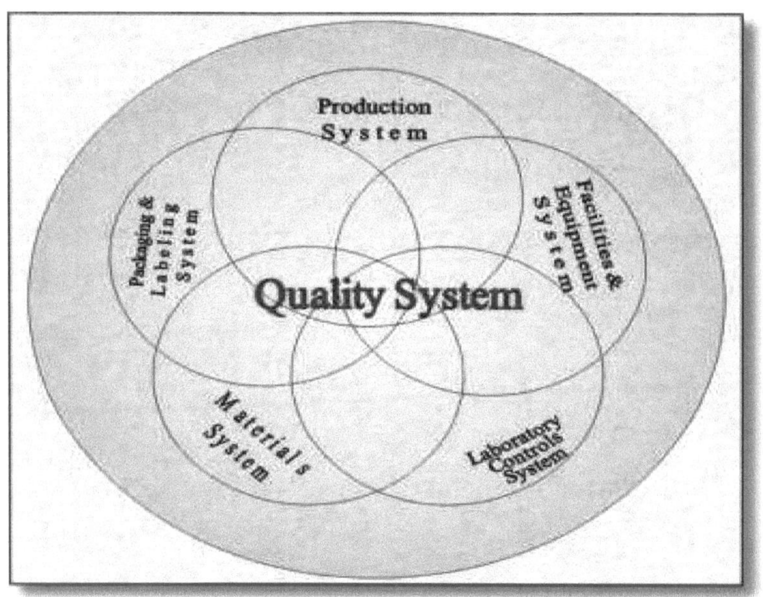

What is the Quality (Control) Unit and What Do They Do?

- Quality control department is responsible for
    - testing the raw materials,
    - in- process samples, intermediates, APIs finished products and
    - the stability samples.

Traditionally the quality of a product was determined only by the testing of the product and determining that it complied with the established specification.

- However the regulatory agency requirement today is that quality is not determined only by end product testing but quality is to built up into the product.
- This entails that at each step quality is to be ensured right from drug development to the finished product manufacturing and sale.

<u>**The role of DQA in case of API - R&D development is to:**</u>

- **1.** To ensure that the raw materials used in the manufacturing are qualified and that all data including the vendor qualification, route of synthesis, declarations are available.

- 2. To ensure that all R&D and analytical development data is recorded by the R&D scientists in laboratory notebooks and is reviewed for accuracy and traceability. This data should be recorded as per the requirements of GMP and should be securely stored/archived for future reference.

- 3. To ensure that the critical process parameters in an API manufacturing process are identified, required testing methods are validated and the R&D batches are initiated for stability.

- 4. To ensure that a system is in place for document control and that procedures are in place for performing the activities, operating and calibrating the equipment and training the personnel.

- In any pharmaceutical company there are a number of departments which are involved in

- the development,

- manufacturing and

- marketing of the drug product

- the R&D,

- purchase,

- production,

- stores,

- engineering,

- QC,

- QA

- As the ICH rightly says: "Quality is the responsibility of all the persons involved in the manufacturing".

The QA department plays an important role throughout the life cycle of the drug substance and drug product and is mentioned as given below:

- MHRA- Medicines and Healthcare products Regulatory Agency
- TGA- Therapeutic Goods Administration
- Brazil and Mexico –Health Authority
- Medicines Control Council (MCC)
- Definitions of Pharmaceutical QualityMany definitions of drug quality exist.
- The pharmaceutical industry has proposed

fitness for use —meaning that the drug meets its pre specified quality attributes or regulatory specifications.

- USP monographs contain compendial assays for evaluating the quality of drugs in the marketplace.
- It has also been stated that a drug manufactured in compliance with CGMPs is a high-quality drug.
- Each of these definitions has certain limitations.
- This practice is intended to ensure that subsequent production batches deliver the same clinical performance as the investigational batches—
    - the dosing,
    - safety, and efficacy as described in the label

So one aspect of the FDA drug quality definition might be:

- delivers clinical performance per label claims.
- A result to this statement is: does not introduce additional risks due to unexpected contaminants
- The Relationships Among Fitness for Use, Quality Attributes and Clinical PerformanceFitness for use has been proposed as such a surrogate definition of pharmaceutical quality.
- A product that is fit for use can be defined as <u>one that meets its established quality attributes and standards and has been manufactured in accordance with CGMP regulations.</u>

Analytical techniques

1.Titrimetric techniques

2. Chromatographic techniques

3. Spectroscopic techniques

4. Fluorimetry and phosphorimetry

5. Electrochemical methods

1. Titrimétric techniques

- With the development of functional group analysis procedures titrimetric methods have been shown to be beneficial in kinetic measurements which are in turn applied to establish reaction rates.

- There are many advantages associated with these methods which include saving time and labor, high precision and the fact that there is no need of using reference standards.

- In addition to its application in drug estimation titrimetric has been used in the past for the estimation of degradation products of the pharmaceuticals.

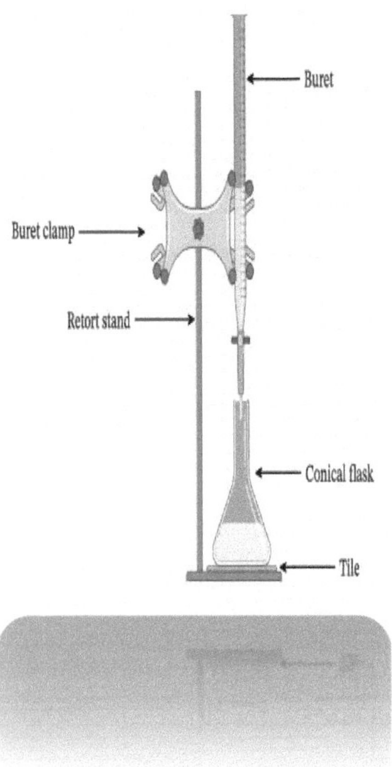

2. Chromatographic techniques

1. Thin layer chromatography

- Thin layer chromatography is a popular technique for the analysis of a wide variety of organic and inorganic materials, because of its distinctive advantages such as
- minimal sample clean-up,
- wide choice of mobile phases,
- flexibility in sample distinction,
- high sample loading capacity and low cost.
- TLC is a powerful tool for <u>screening unknown materials in bulk drugs</u>.

- TLC plays a crucial role in the early stage of drug development when information about the impurities and degradation products in drug substance and drug product is inadequate.
- Various impurities of pharmaceuticals have been identified and determined using TLC

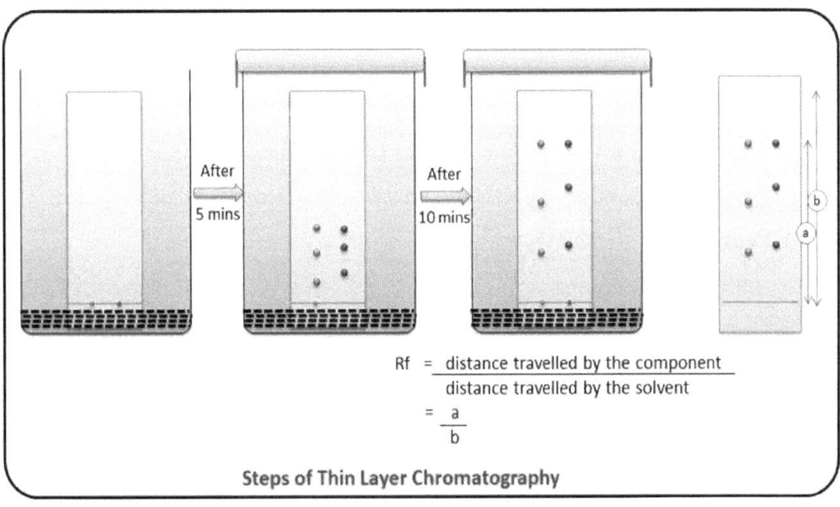

Steps of Thin Layer Chromatography

2. High performance thin layer chromatography

- HPTLC is a fast separation technique and flexible enough to analyze a wide variety of samples.

- This technique is advantageous in many means as it is simple to handle and requires a short analysis time to analyze the complex or the crude sample cleanup.
- HPTLC evaluates the entire chromatogram with a variety of parameters without time limits. Moreover, there is simultaneous but independent development of multiple samples and standards on each plate, leading to an increased reliability of results

3. High-performance liquid chromatography (HPLC)

- HPLC is an advanced form of liquid chromatography used in separating the complex mixture of molecules encountered in chemical and biological systems, in order to recognize better the role of individual molecules.
- Among the chromatographic techniques HPLC has been the most widely used system

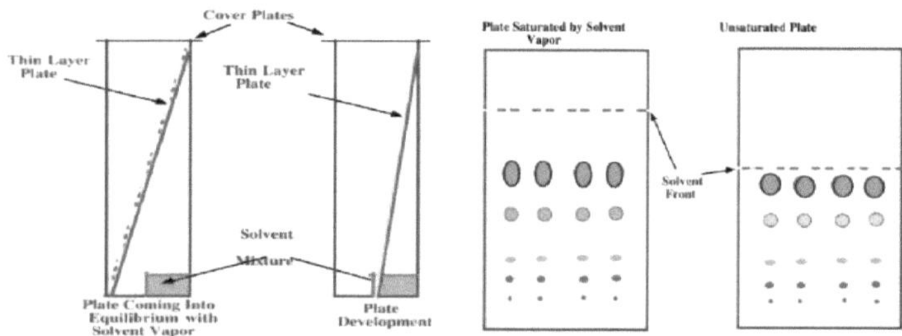

4. Gas chromatography

- Gas chromatography is a powerful separation technique for detection of volatile organic compounds.
- Combining separation and on-line detection allows accurate quantitative determination of complex mixtures, including traces of compounds down to parts per trillions in some specific cases.
- Gas liquid chromatography commands a substantial role in the analysis of pharmaceutical product
- The creation of high-molecular mass products such as polypeptides, or thermally unstable antibiotics confines the scope of this technique.

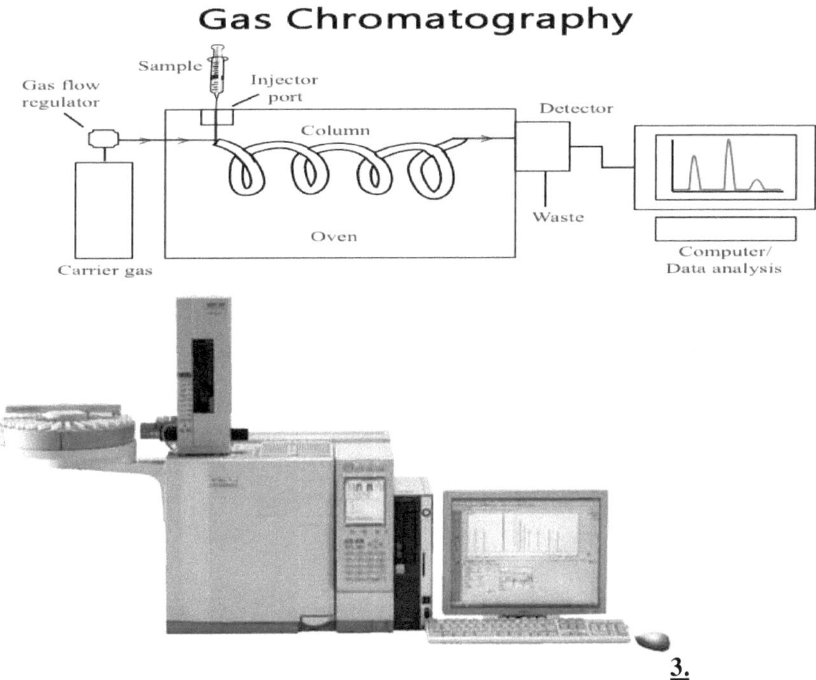

<u>**Spectroscopic techniques**</u>
- 1. Spectrophotometry

- Another important group of methods which find an important place in pharmacopoeias are spectrophotometric <u>methods based on natural UV absorption and chemical reactions</u> .

- Spectrophotometry is the <u>quantitative measurement</u> of the reflection or transmission properties of a material as a function of wavelength.

- The advantages of these methods are <u>low time and labor consumption</u>. The precision of these methods is also excellent. The use of UV–Vis spectrophotometry especially applied in the analysis of pharmaceutical dosage form has increased rapidly over the last few years.

- The colorimetric methods are usually based on the following aspects:
    - *Complex-formation reaction.*
    - *Oxidation-reduction process.*
    - *A catalytic effect.*

- It is important to mention that <u>colorimetric methods are regularly used for the</u> <u>assay of bulk materials.</u>

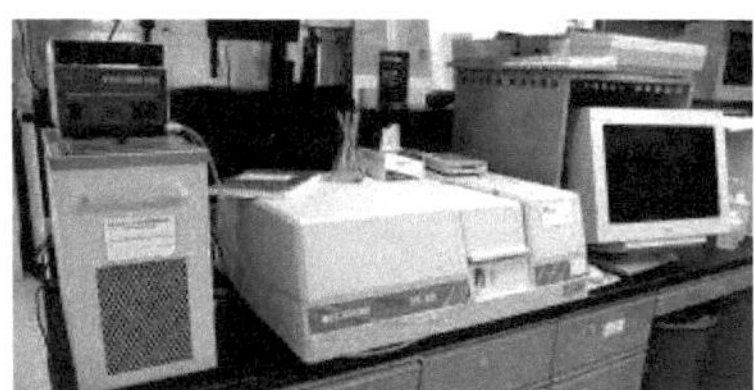

2. Near infrared spectroscopy (NIRS)

■ Near infrared spectroscopy (NIRS) is a rapid and nondestructive procedure that provides multi component analysis of almost any matrix.

■ In recent years, NIR spectroscopy has gained a wide appreciation within the pharmaceutical industry for raw material testing, product quality control and process monitoring.

■ The growing pharmaceutical interest in NIR spectroscopy is probably a direct consequence of its major advantages over other analytical techniques, namely, an easy sample preparation without any pretreatments, the probability of separating the sample measurement position by use of fiber optic probes, and the expectation of chemical and physical sample parameters from one single spectrum.

3. Nuclear magnetic resonance spectroscopy (NMR)

■ Recently NMR finds its application in quantitative analysis in order to determine the impurity of the drugcharacterization of the composition of the drug products and in quantitation of drugs in pharmaceutical formulations and biological fluids.

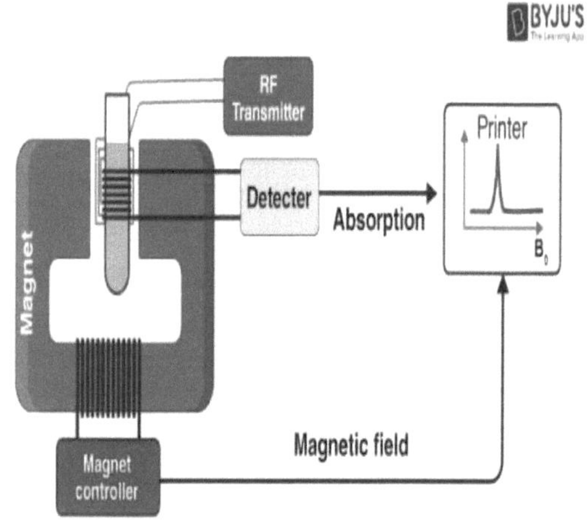

NMR Spectroscopy Instrumentation

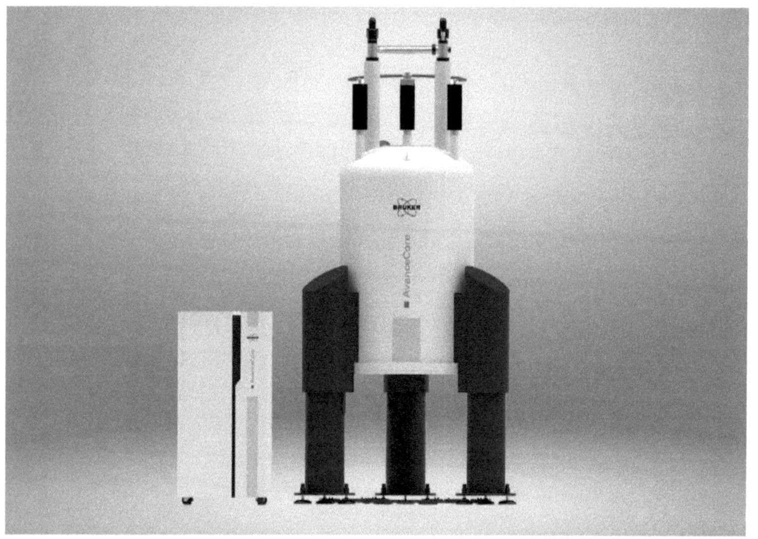

4. Fluorimetry and phosphorimetry

- The pharmaceutical industries continuously look for the sensitive analytical techniques using the micro samples.

- Fluorescence spectrometry is one of the techniques that serve the purpose of high sensitivity without the loss of specificity or precision

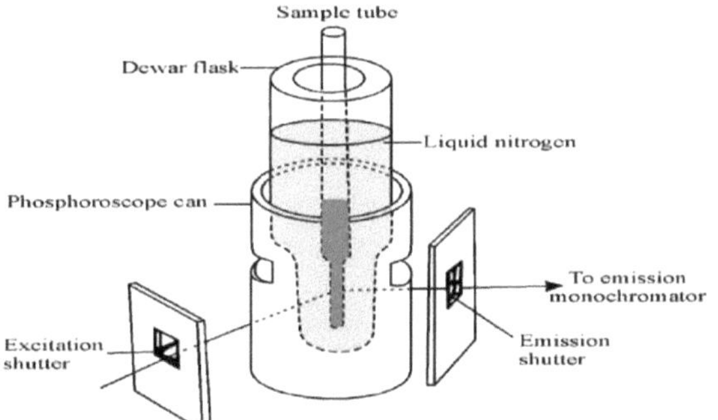

Fig. 5.9: Revolving can shutter system for recording phosphorescence and fluorescence from the same sample

5. Electrochemical methods

- The application of electrochemical techniques in the analysis of drugs and pharmaceuticals has increased greatly over the last few years.

- The renewed interest in electrochemical techniques can be attributed in part to more sophisticated instrumentation and to increase the understanding of the technique themselves.

Technique

- Voltammetry
- Polarography
- Amperometry
- Potentiometry

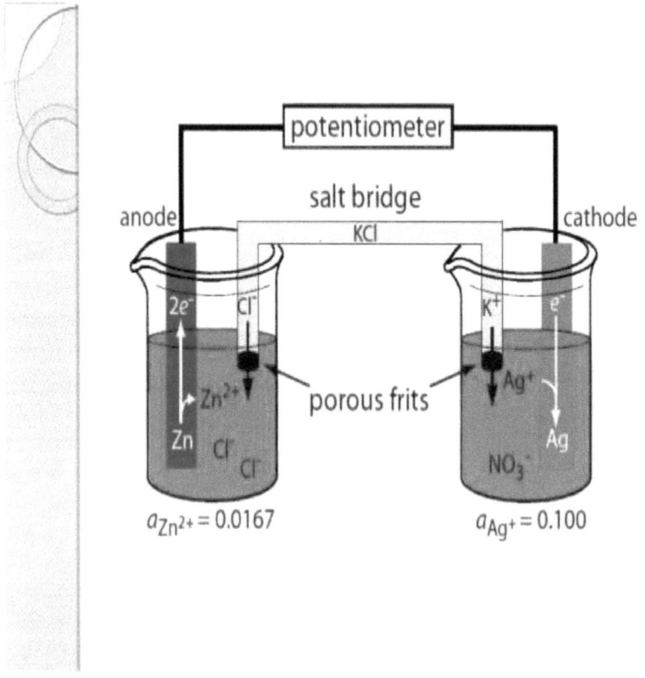

Impurities in pharmaceutical products.

- Impurity: Any component of the new drug substance that is <u>not the chemical entity</u> or is an <u>unwanted chemical.</u>

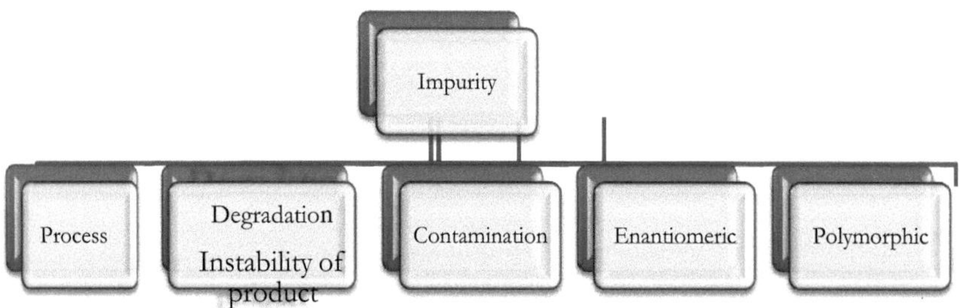

Sources of impurities in drug products

- Raw materials

- Method of manufacture adopted
- Instability of the product
- Atmospheric contaminants

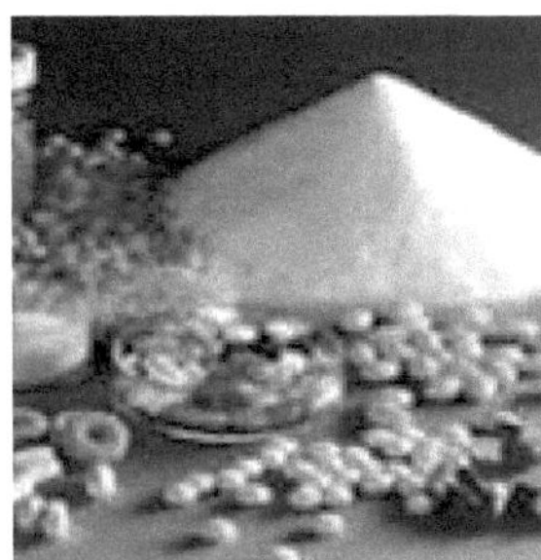
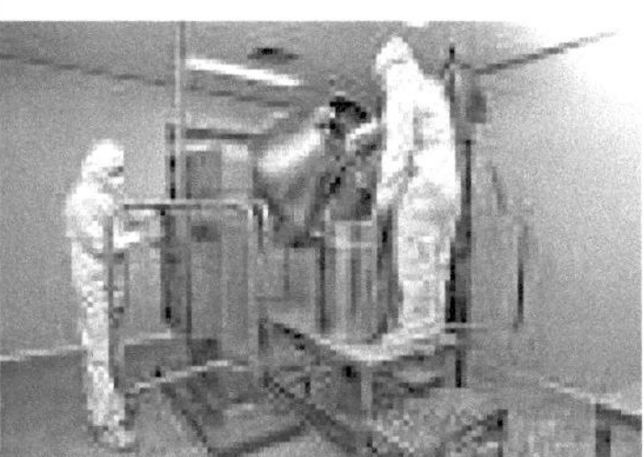

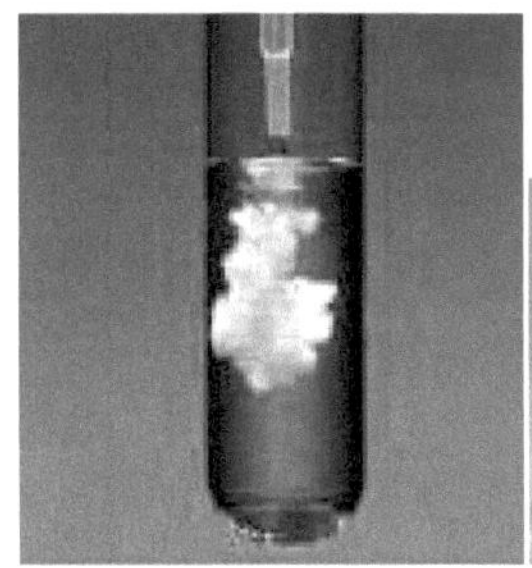
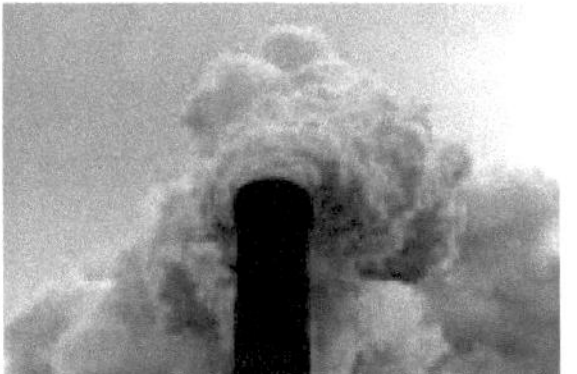

Sources of impurities in drug products

- Method of manufacture
  - *Reagents*
  - *Solvents*
  - *Reaction vessels*

49

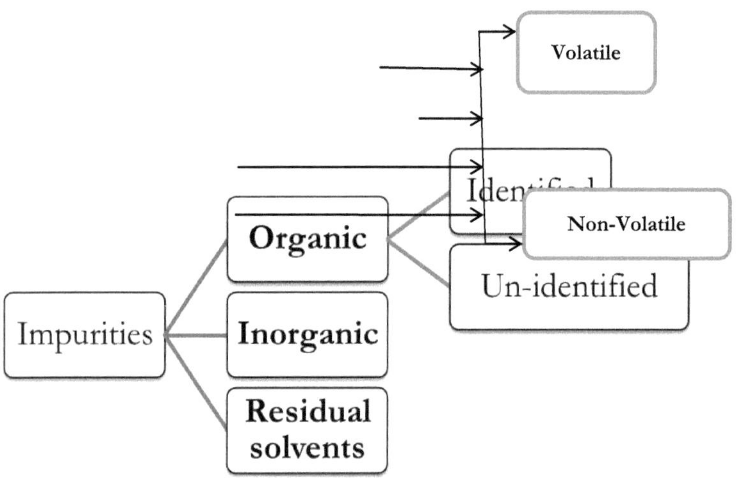

Classification of impurities

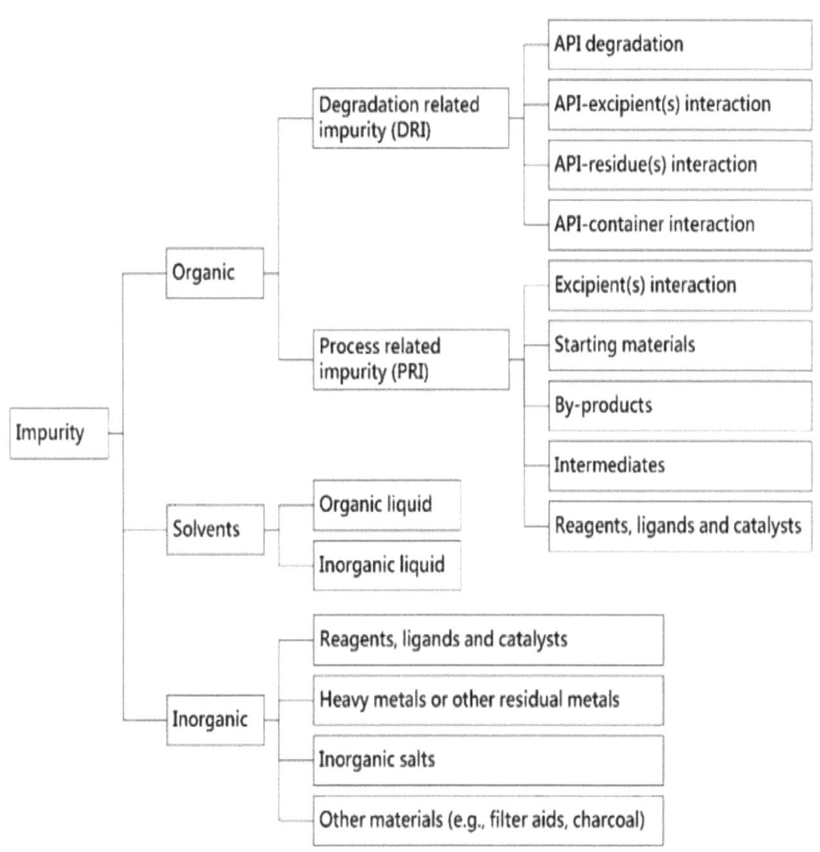

Regulatory requirements for the management of impurity

Impurities	Drug substances	Drug products	Biological products
Organic impurities: Process-related	ICH Q3A, FDA 2009, USP <1086>	USP <1086>	WHO 2014 (Series No. 987)
Organic impurities: Drug-related products		ICH Q3B, FDA 2010	
Residual solvents	ICH Q3C, USP <467>		ICH Q3C*
Inorganic & elemental	ICH Q3D, USP <232>, <233>, <1086>, EMA 2007, 2008, 2017		
		FDA 2018	
Genotoxic	FDA 2008		
	ICH M7		
	EMA 2006		

Learning outcomes

- After the completion of unit, students will be able to:

1. Explain various concepts in quality control

2. Assess the idea of quality assurance

3. Explain various concepts in Analytical techniques in pharmaceutical analysis

4. Draw conclusions from the analytical reports

5. Explain sources of impurities in pharmaceutical products.

CHAPTER 3

Evaluation of Pharmaceutical Tablets

Evaluation of Pharmaceutical Tablets

<u>Objectives:</u>

1. To describe pharmaceutical tablets dosage form.

2. To know the In Process Quality Control Tests (IPQC) for Pharmaceutical tablets

3. To perform Official and Unofficial Tests for Evaluation of Tablets.

Pharmaceutical tablets dosage form.

- Tablets are solid preparations each containing a single dose of one or more active ingredients.
- prepared by <u>compression</u> although some tablets are prepared by moulding. <u>Cavity plate and peg plate</u>

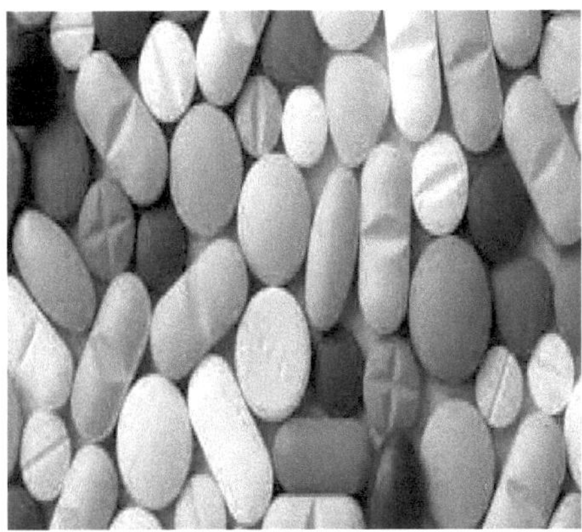

> Many different types of tablets are available, which may be in a variety of shapes and sizes.

These include

> dispersible or effervescent,

> chewable,

> sublingual and buccal tablets,

> lozenges,

> tablets for vaginal administration and

> solution tablets.

> Some tablets are designed to release the medication slowly for prolonged drug release and sustained drug action.

> In addition to the active ingredient, several excipients, or inactive ingredients are added.

> These aid the process of tableting and ensure that the active ingredients are released in the body as intended.

Excipients include

1. Diluents or fillers:

These add bulk to make the tablet easier to handle.
Examples include lactose, mannitol, microcrystalline cellulose and calcium carbonate.

2. Binders or adhesives:

These enable granules to be prepared which <u>improve flow properties</u> of the mixture and compression.

Examples include
 acacia, mucilage, glucose, povidone and starch mucilage.

3. Disintegrators or disintegrating agents.
These ensure that the tablet breaks down into its component particles after ingestion.
Examples include sodium alginate, carmellose sodium, microcrystalline cellulose, sodium glycin carbonate and starch.

4. Antiadherents, glidants, lubricants or lubricating agents:

-Lubricants are essential for flow of the tablet material into the tablet dies and preventing sticking of the compressed tablet in the punch and die.

 Examples of lubricants are magnesium and calcium stearate, sodium lauryl sulphate and sodium stearyl fumarate.

-Colloidal silica is usually the glidant of choice.

-Talc and magnesium stearate are effective antiadherents.

5. Miscellaneous agents may be added, such as colours and flavours in chewable tablets.

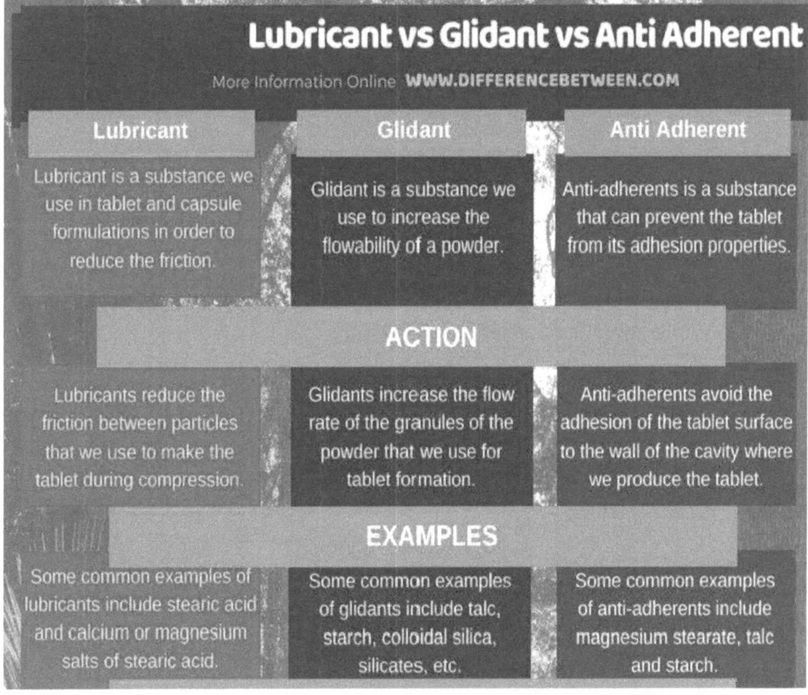

Lubricant	Glidant

Pharmaceutical Application	To smooth ejection of tablet from die cavity by reducing inter-particle friction.	To improve powder flow

Pharmaceutical tablets testing:

Official Tests

[1] Weight variation

[2] Disintegration

[3] Dissolution

[4] Drug content

Non-Official Tests

[1] Hardness

[2] Friability

Physical Appearance:

- The general appearance of a tablet, its identity and general elegance is essential for consumer acceptance, for control of lot-to-lot uniformity and tablet-to-tablet uniformity.
- The control of general appearance involves the measurement of size, shape, color, presence or absence of odor, taste etc.
  Weight variation

Weight variation

- Weigh individually 20 units selected at random and calculate the average weight.
- Not more than two of the individual weights deviate from the average weight by more than the percentage shown in the table and none deviates by more than twice that percentage

Weight Variation Tolerances for Uncoated Tablet

Sr. no	Average wt. of tablet(mg)	Max. % difference allowed
1	130 or Less	10%
2	130-324	7.5%
3	More than 324	5%

Sr. no	Average wt. of tablet(mg)	Max. % difference allowed
1	84 or Less	10%
2	84-250	7.5%
3	More than 250	5%

Content Uniformity Test

> The test for uniformity of content of single-dose preparations is based on the assay of the individual contents of active substance(s) of a number of single-dose units to determine whether the individual contents are within limits set with reference to the average content of the sample

› **Method:** Determine the content of active ingredient(s) in each of 10 dosage units taken at random using the method given in the monograph or by any other suitable analytical method.

› **Acceptance limits for tablets, suspensions for injection and ophthalmic inserts:** The preparation complies with the test if each individual content is 85-115 % of average content.

› Randomly select 30 tablets.

› 10 of these assayed individually.

› The Tablet pass the test if 9 of the 10 tablets must contain not less than 85 % and not more than 115 % of the labeled drug content and the 10th tablet may not contain less than 75 % and more than125 % of the labeled content.

› If these conditions are not met, remaining 20 tablet assayed individually and none may fall outside of the 85 to 115 % range.

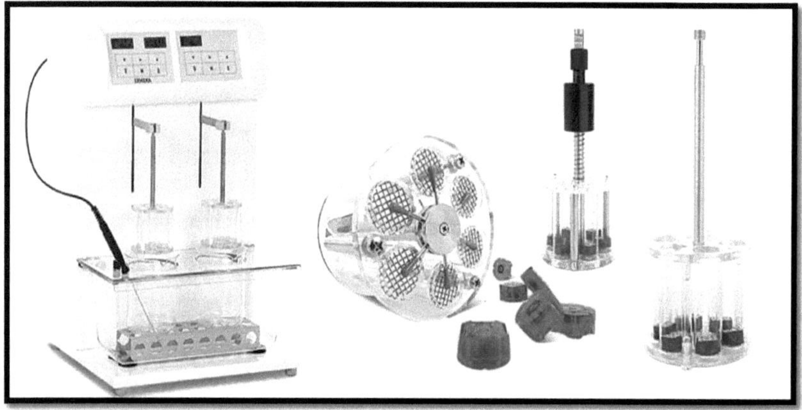

Sr. no	Type of tablets	Medium	Temperature	limit
1	Compressed uncoated		$37 \pm 2\ ^0C$	<u>15 minutes</u> or as per individual monograph
2	Sugar coated	If 1 or 2 tablets fail Water 0.1 N HCL	$37 \pm 2\ ^0C$	<u>60 minutes</u> or as per individual monograph
3	Film coated	water	$37 \pm 2\ ^0C$	30 minutes or as per individual monograph
4	Enteric coated	0.1 N HCL & Phosphate buffer pH 6.8	$37 \pm 2\ ^0C$	<u>1 hr</u> or as per individual monograph
5	Dispersible/ Effervescent	water	$37 \pm 2\ ^0C$	< 3 minutes or as per individual monograph
6	Buccal		$37 \pm 2\ ^0C$	**4 hr** or as per individual monograph

U.S.P. and B.P Method for Enteric coated tablets :

> Put in distilled water for <u>five minutes to dissolve the coat.</u>

> Then put in simulated <u>gastric fluid (0.1M HCL) for one hour.</u>

> Then put in simulated intestinal fluid for two hours.

> If one or two tablets fail to disintegrate, repeat this test on another 12 tablets.

> So 16 tablets from 18 should completely disintegrate.

> If more than two fail to disintegrate the Batch must be rejected

Dissolution test

› Dissolution is mass transfer process.

› n Dissolution is mainly depend on aqueous solubility of drug.

› n It is process in which solid mass transfer in liquid medium. n Dissolution based on four process –

› 1. wetting 2. Solubility 3. Swelling 4. Diffusion.

› n <u>Particle size, shape, surface area</u> is important factor can affect the <u>rate of dissolution</u> of drug.

› n The aqueous solubility is increases, increases rate of dissolution drug

Dissolution test apparatus

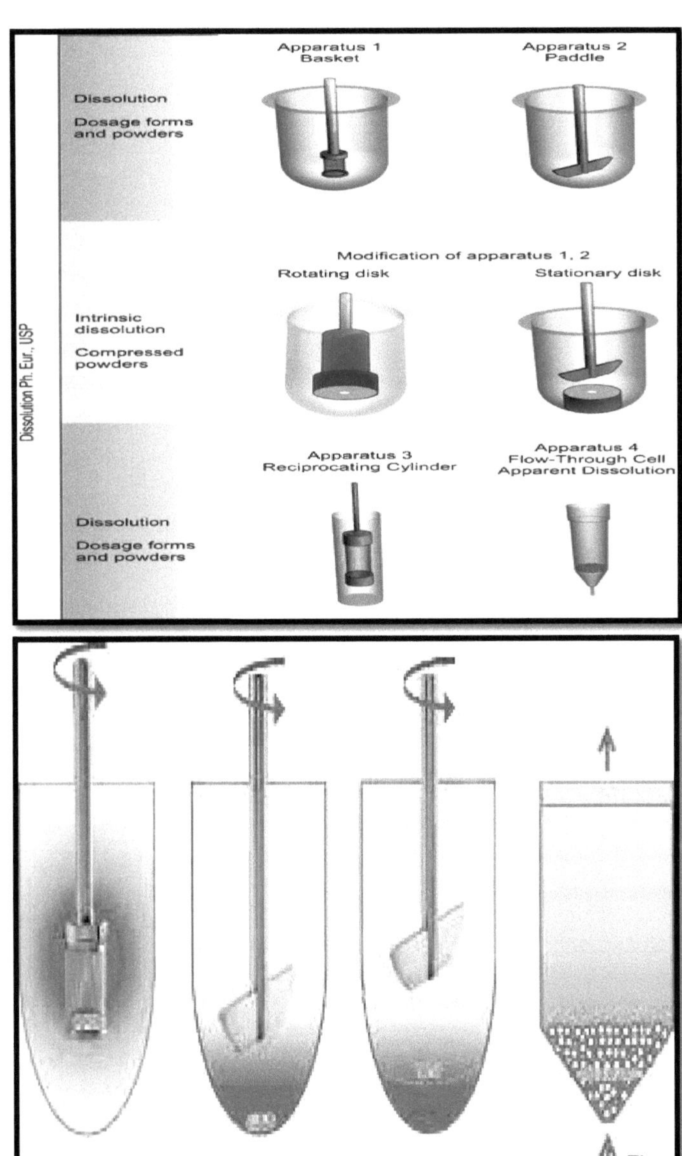

Dissolution Ph. Eur., USP
Apparatus 1
Basket
Apparatus 2
Paddle
Dissolution
Dosage forms
and powders
Modification of apparatus 1, 2
Rotating disk
Stationary disk
Intrinsic
dissolution
Compressed
powders
Apparatus 3
Reciprocating Cylinder
Apparatus 4
Flow-Through Cell
Apparent Dissolution
Dissolution
Dosage forms
and powders
Flow

Dissolution test apparatus

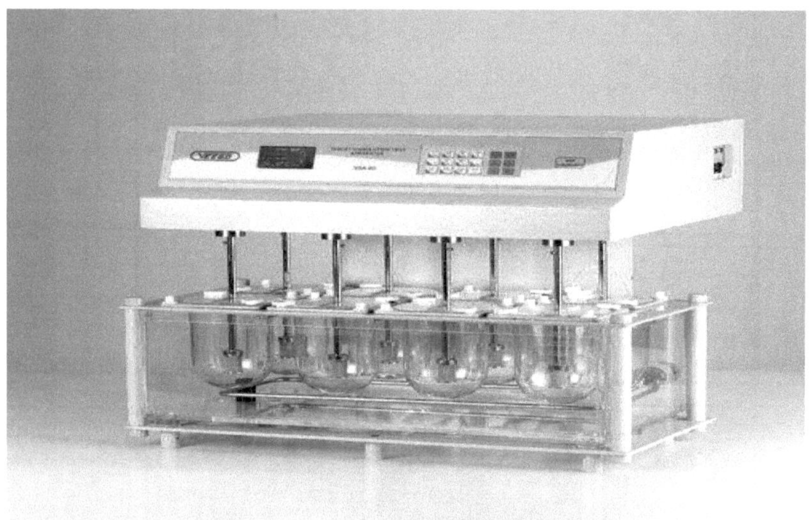

d) Dissolution test apparatus :

> Dissolution test apparatus IP apparatus [1] First is Paddle apparatus (IP) [2] Second is Basket apparatus (IP)

> USP apparatus

> 1. Apparatus 1 (rotating basket)

> 2. Apparatus 2 (paddle assembly)

> 3. Apparatus 3 (reciprocating cylinder)

> 4. Apparatus 4 (flow-through cell)

> 5. Apparatus 5 (paddle over disk)

> 6. Apparatus 6 (cylinder)

> 7. Apparatus 7 (reciprocating holder)

Dissolution test- Immediate release tablet (conventional tablet)

> 1. Dissolution apparatus – Type 1 and Type 2 (USP)

> 2. Temperature - 37±0.5°C

› 3. Time – 30 min

› 4. Time of interval – 5, 10, 15, 20, 25, 30.

› 5. Media – PH 1.2 Acidic Buffer, PH 4.5 Acetate buffer, PH 5.8 Phosphate buffer.

› (depending upon tablet)

› 6. Rpm – 75 -100 rpm

› 7. Volume – 900 ml

Dissolution test Procedure:

› The tablet was added into cylindrical vessel containing 1000 ml dissolution media having rpm 75 and tem.37±0.5°C.

› Dissolution of tablet was conducted 30 min, in 5 min. of interval, after 5 min 5 mL sample was removed and appropriate quantity of sample take absorbance by using U.V. spectroscopy technique and determine <u>rate of dissolution of tablet.</u>

› Dissolution test: Sustained release tablet Sustained release tablet

› 1. Dissolution apparatus – Type 2 (USP)

› 2. Temperature - 37±0.5°C

› 3. Time – 7 hrs

› 4. Media – PH 1.2 Acidic Buffer, PH 6.8 Phosphate buffer.

› 5. Rpm – 75 – 100.

› 6. Volume – 900 ml.

› Dissolution test: Sustained release tablet Procedure - The tablet was added into cylindrical vessel containing 1000 ml PH 1.2 Acidic media having rpm 75 for next two hours and tem. 37±0.5°C.

› Dissolution media was changes tablet was added in to PH 6.8 Phosphate buffer for <u>next five hour </u>for 1 hr. of interval.

> After 1 hr. 5 mL sample was removed and appropriate quantity of sample take absorbance by using U.V. spectroscopy technique and determine rate of dissolution of tablet.

Hardness Test

Importance

> To determine the need for pressure adjustments on the tableting machine.

> Hardness can affect the disintegration.

> So if the tablet is too hard, it may not disintegrate in the required period of time.

> And if the tablet is too soft, it will not withstand the handling during subsequent processing such as coating or packaging.

> In general, if the tablet hardness is too high, we first check its disintegration before rejecting the batch.

> If the disintegration is within limit, we accept the batch.

> If Hardness is high + disintegration is within a time accept the batch.

> Hardness Test**(i) By Manual Testing**: Manual testing method was employed previously. In this, method, the thumb acts as a fulcrum, while the tablet is held between the second and third hand fingers. When the pressure is applied the tablet which breaks with a sharp snap deemed to posses' sufficient hardness.

> **(ii) Monsanto Hardness Tester Method :**

> The instrument measures the force required to break the tablet when the force generated by a coil spring is applied diametrically to the tablet.

> (Iii) **Pfizer Hardness Tester**: Force required to break tablet is recorded on dial and may be expressed in key pounds

> **Other devices**:
> · Strong-Cobb Hardness Tester
> · Erweka Hardness Tester.
> · Schleuniger or Heberlein Hardness Tester.
> **Acceptance criteria**: <u>**A force of 4 kg is considered to be the minimum requirement for a satisfactory tablet.**</u>

Schleuniger type

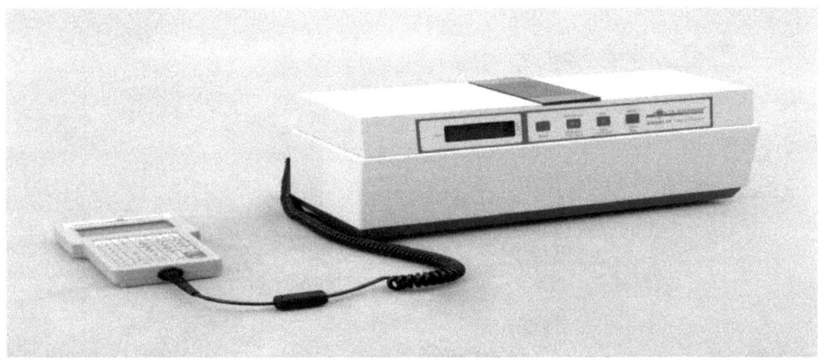

Friability

> Friability of a tablet can determine in laboratory by Roche friabilator.

> This consist of a plastic chamber that revolves at 25 rpm, dropping the tablets through a Distance of six inches in the friabilator, which is then operate for 100 revolutions.

> The tablets are reweighed.

> A maximum loss of weight (from a single test or from the mean of the three tests) not greater than 1.0 per cent is acceptable for most tablets.

> If obviously cracked, chipped or broken tablets are present in the sample after tumbling, the sample fails the test.

> This test is applicable to compressed tablets and is intended to determine the physical strength of tablets.

Learning Outcomes

> After completing this chapter, students can able to explain

> In Process Quality Control Tests (IPQC) for Pharmaceutical tablets and to perform Official and Unofficial Tests for Evaluation of Tablets.

CHAPTER-4

Quality Standards and Compendial Requirements for capsules

Evaluation of Pharmaceutical Capsules

<u>Objectives:</u>

1. To describe pharmaceutical capsules dosage form.
2. To evaluate capsules dosage form

Pharmaceutical capsules dosage form

<u>CAPSULES :</u>

- Capsules are solid dosage forms in which medicinal agents are enclosed in <u>small shell of Gelatin</u>.
- Capsule shells may be <u>hard</u> or <u>soft,</u> depending on their composition.

<u>a) Physical appearance:</u>

- The general appearance of a capsule, its identity and general elegance is essential for consumer acceptance, for control of lot-to-lot uniformity and capsule uniformity.
- The control of general appearance involves the measurement of size, shape, color, presence or absence of odor and taste.

<u>**b) Weight variation test:**</u>

- Weigh an intact capsule.
- Open it without losing any part of the shell and remove the contents as completely as possible.
- For <u>soft gelatin capsules,</u> <u>wash the shell</u> with a suitable solvent and keep aside until the odour of the solvent is not perceptible.
- <u>Weigh the shell.</u>
- The <u>difference between the weighing gives the weight of the contents.</u>
- Repeat the procedure with another 19 capsules If not, they must be sealed by moistening the outside top of the body before putting the top in place.

<u>**c) Uniformity of content:**</u>

- The preparation complies with the test if not more than one individual content is outside the limits of 85-115% of the average content and none is outside the limits of 75-125 %of the average content.
- The preparation <u>fails to comply with the test if more than three individual contents are outside the limits of 85-115%</u> of the average content or if one or more individual contents are outside the limits of 75- 125 % of the avg content.
- If <u>two or three individual contents are outside the limits of 85-115%</u> of the average content but within the limits of 75-125%, repeat the determination using another 20 dosage units.
- The preparation complies with the test if not more than 3 individual contents of the total sample of 30 dosage units are outside the limits of 85-115 per cent of the average content and none is outside the limits of 75-125 %of the average content.

<u>d) Closing length:</u>

- The Acceptance criteria 0.2mm

<u>e) Moisture permeation test:</u>

- To assure the suitability of containers for packaging
- capsules, USP has started some rules and regulations.
- According those rules and regulations, the moisture
- permeating feature of capsules packaged in single unit
- containers is to be determined.

Procedure:

- For performing this test, one capsule is packaged along with the dehydrated pellets, which have the property of changing colour in the presence moisture.
- The packaged capsule is then placed for a certain period of time in an atmosphere of known humidity.
- <u>Any change in the colour of dehydrated pellets reveals the absorption of moisture.</u>
- The weight of this capsule is then compared with the weights of the capsules under test.
- The differences in the weights give the amount of moisture absorbed

MOISTURE PERMEATION TEST

The degree and rate of moisture penetration is determined by packaging the dosage unit together with a colour revealing desiccant pellet

⇩

Expose the packed unit to known relative humidity over a specified time

⇩

Observe the desiccant pellet for colour change

⇩

Any change in colour indicates absorption of moisture

⇩

By measuring pre test weight and protest weight of pellet, amount can be calculated.

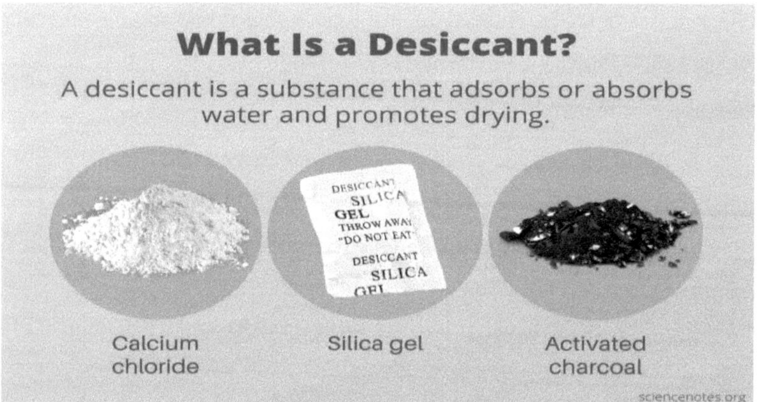

CHAPTER 5

Evaluation of Liquid Dosage forms

Evaluation of the oral liquid preparations

OBJECTIVE

- ➡ To Know the Quality Control Tests for evaluation of the oral liquid preparations
- ➡ To Know the Quality Control Tests for evaluation Syrups, Elixirs and Tinctures
- ➡ To Know the Quality Control Tests for evaluation of the oral Suspension
- ➡ To Know the Quality Control Tests for evaluation of the oral Emulsion

What are LIQUID DOSAGE FORMS?

- It is prepared by dissolving active ingredients or by suspending the drug (if drug is insoluble) or by incorporating the drug into one of the two phases of oil and water systems.

i) Monophasic

- a) Syrups,
- b) Elixirs,
- c) Tinctures

(ii) Biphasic

- a) Suspensions
- b) Emulsions

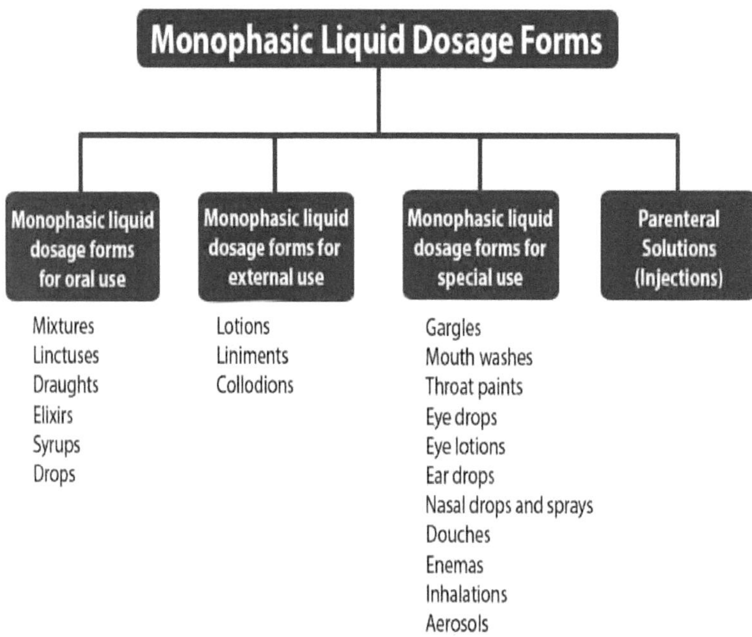

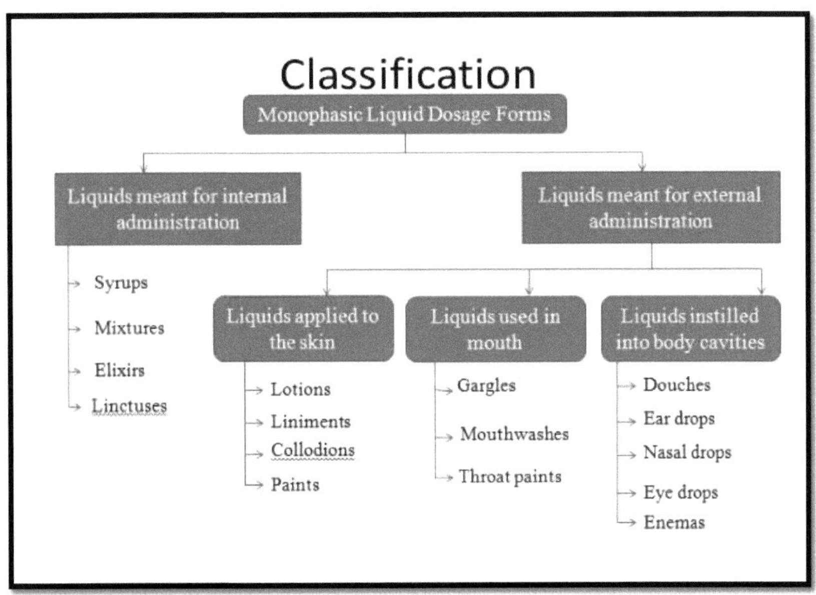

Classification
Monophasic Liquid Dosage Forms
Liquids meant for internal administration
Liquids meant for external administration
Syrups
Mixtures
Elixirs
Linctuses
Liquids applied to the skin
Lotions
Liniments
Collodions
Paints
Liquids used in mouth
Gargles
Mouthwashes
Throat paints
Liquids instilled into body cavities
Douches
Ear drops
Nasal drops
Eye drops
Enemas

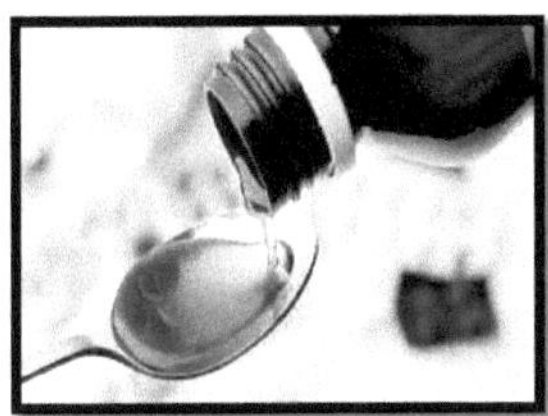

LIQUID DOSAGE FORMS

- Liquid dosage form comprises of solution, suspension and emulsion and a variety of preparation can be considered under each category.
- These dosage form are categorized by their homogenies, promote action and easy of Administration.
- Liquid dosage forms are suitable for both internal and external use.
- This is a general term used to describe a solution, suspension or emulsion in which the active ingredient is dissolved or dispersed in a suitable liquid vehicle.

IPQC TESTS FOR MONOPHASIC LIQUID DOSAGE FORMS:

- a) Uniformity of content
- b) Uniformity of Weight / Volume
- c) Leakage Test

IPQC TESTS FOR MONOPHASIC LIQUID DOSAGE FORMS:

a) Uniformity of content:

- Unless otherwise specified, single dose liquids in suspension form and that contain less than 10 mg or less than 10 per cent of active ingredient complies with the following test.
- For oral liquids containing more than one active ingredient carry out the test for each active ingredient that corresponds to the above conditions.

Uniformity of content

Method:

- Determine the content of active ingredient(s) of each of 10 containers taken at random, using the method given in the monograph or by any other suitable analytical method of equivalent accuracy and precision.
- The preparation under examination complies with the test if the individual values thus obtained are all between 85-115% of the average value.
- The preparation under examination fails to comply with the test if more than one individual value is outside the limits 85-115% of the average value or if any one individual value is outside the limits 75-125 % of the average value.

Uniformity of content

- If one individual value is outside the limits 85-115 % but within the limits 75-125% of the average value, repeat the determination using another 20 containers taken at random.
- The preparation under examination complies with the test if in the total sample of 30 contains not more than one individual value is outside the limits 85 -115 % and none is outside the limits 75 -125 % of the average value.

b) Uniformity of Weight/Volume

- The following tests and specifications apply to oral dosage forms and preparations intended for topical use that are packaged in containers in which the labelled net quantity is <u>not more than 100 g or 300 ml or 1000 units,</u> as the case may be.
- For higher labelled quantities the test and limits given in the standards of Weights and Measures (Packaged commodities) Rules, may be followed

c) Leakage Test

- Ampoules are subjected to leakage test because ampoules are sealed by fusion.
- Therefore, there is a chance for a incomplete sealing or for microspores to exist, allowing the contents to leak or microorganisms and other contaminants to enter the ampoules.

c) Leakage Test Method:

- This test is performed by immersing the ampoules in a vacuum chamber consisting of a dye such as 1% methylene blue solution.
- A vacuum (negative pressure) of about 27 inch Hg or more is created for about 15 to 30 minutes.
- This negative pressure causes the methylene blue solution to enter the ampoules with defective sealing.

- The vacuum is released, ampoules are washed externally and observed for the presence of dye in the ampoules.
- The colored solution because of the dye in the ampoules confirms the leakage and hence those ampoules are discarded.

(ii) BIPHASIC LIQUID DOSAGE FORMS

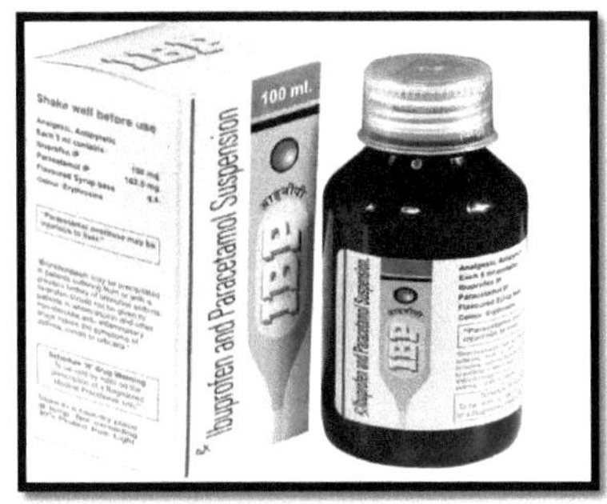

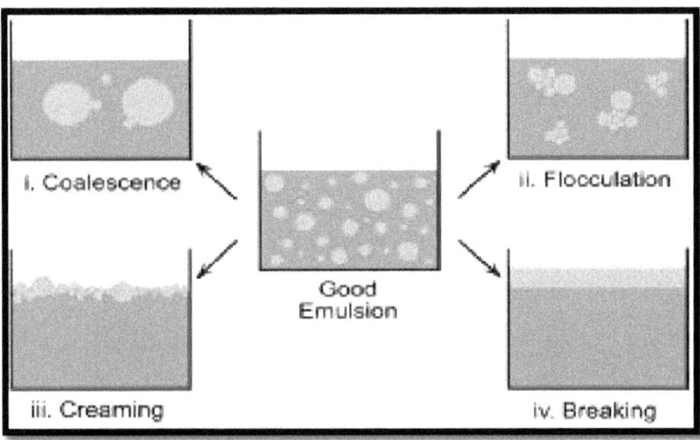
i. Coalescence
ii. Flocculation
Good
Emulsion
iii. Creaming
iv. Breaking

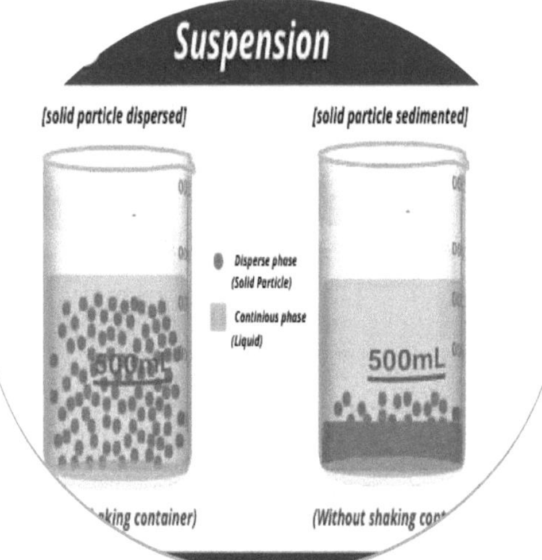

- **IPQC TESTS FOR BIPHASIC LIQUID DOSAGE FORMS**:
- a) Appearance:
- c) Determination of Particle Size
- d) Uniformity of Volume
- b) Color, Odor and Taste:
- e) Viscosity
- F) Density
- g) Degree of Flocculation
- h) Extent of Sedimentation
- i)Redispersibility
- j) Zeta potential

ii) BIPHASIC LIQUID DOSAGE FORMS

a) Suspensions:

- ➡ Pharmaceutical suspensions may be defined as coarse dispersions in which insoluble solids are suspended in liquid medium.

IPQC tests for suspensions

a) Appearance:

- ➡ The appearance of the suspension is noted and determined the uniformity of sedimentation and also determined the breaks or air pockets in the sediment.

Method:

- ➡ The appearance is noted in a graduated glass cylinder or transparent glass container.
- ➡ Photo microscopic Examination: The microscope can be used to distinguish between flocculated and non-flocculated particles and to determine changes in the physical properties and stability.
- ➡ Sufficient fields and samples should be examined to make these determinations.

Method:

- ➡ Microscope can be used to estimate and detect change in particle size distribution and crystal shape of suspension.

- The dilution of suspension for microscopic examination should be made with supernatant external phase rather than with purified water.
- Individual particle size distributions can be accurately determined, using Suitable electron instrumentation, for example, a Coulter Multisizer II or the Elzone 280 PC systems .

b) Color, Odor and Taste:

- These characteristics are especially important in orally administered suspensions.
- Variation in color Photomicrograph of a flocculated steroid suspension indicates poor distribution and/or differences in particle size.
- Variations in taste, especially of active constituents, can often be attributed to changes in particle size, crystal habit, and subsequent particle dissolution.
- Changes in color, odor, and taste can also indicate chemical instability

b) Color, Odor and Taste:

Method:

- By visualization as product and by testing the drug products pH Value as the presence of H+ ions in the suspension preparation.
- The pH value of aqueous suspensions should be taken at a given temperature and only after settling equilibrium has been reached, to minimize ''pH drift'' and electrode surface coating with suspended particles.

- Immerse the electrodes in the solution under examination and measure the pH at $25° \pm 2°$ (pH range:-4.5- 7.2)

c) Determination of Particle volume:

Coulter counters method:

- This electronic method is used to detect the particles and also determine the Particle volume.
- The sample solution is added to an electrolyte solution.
- This solution is drawn through a small orifice of the device.
- Positive and negative electrodes are present one on either side of an orifice.
- As the particle passes through the orifice, it displaces its own volume of electrolyte and at the same moment, an increase in electrical resistance is observed between the two electrodes.
- The resulting voltage pulses which are proportional to the particle volume, are amplified and are measured and counted.

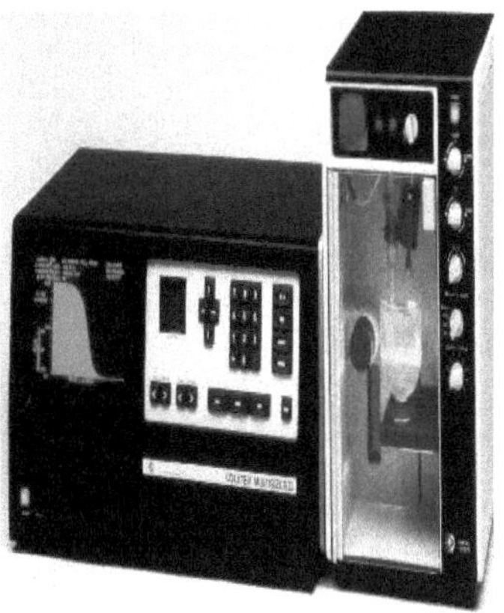

Significance of Particulate Matter Detection:

- The presence of foreign particles in intravenous solutions may cause obstruction of small blood vessels leading to severe consequences like emboli, infusion, and infusion phlebitis ((inflammation of the vein).
- The presence of particulate matter implies that the product is of inferior quality

Microscopic count method (or) membrane filtration method A measured sample solution is filtered through a membrane filter.

- The collected particles on the surface of the filter are then counted with the

  help of a microscope at 100X magnification.
- The whole method is carried out under aseptic conditions. However,

it is a time consuming process.

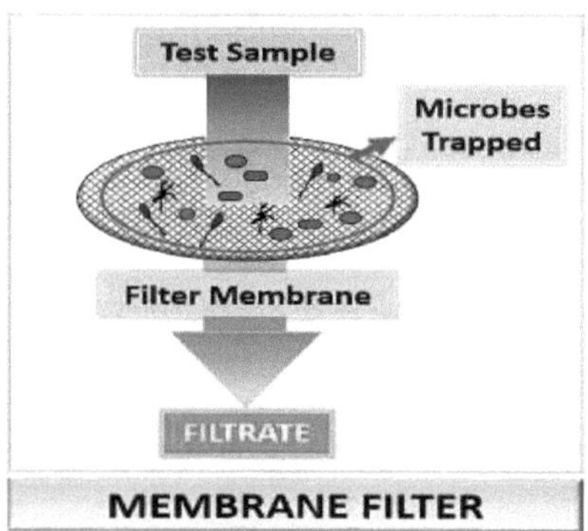

d) Uniformity of Volume

- Pour completely the contents of each container into calibrated volume measures of the appropriate size and determine the volume of the contents of the 10 containers.

d) Uniformity of Volume

Acceptance Criteria: The given % allowance for uniformity of volume according to Pharmacopea:

- If this requirement is not met, test is done on 10 additional containers.
- The average net volume of the contents of the 20 containers is not less than the labelled amount, and
- the net volume of the contents of not more than of the 20 containers is less than 91 per cent or more than 109 per cent of the labelled amount where the labelled amount is 50 ml or less (or) less than 97.0 per cent or more than 103 per cent of the labelled amount where the labelled amount is more than 50 ml but not more than 2oo ml

e) Viscosity:

- A Brookfield viscometer is a useful rheological instrument for measuring the settling behavior and structure of pharmaceutical suspensions and for characterizing the properties sand stability of flocculated suspensions.
- The viscometer should be properly calibrated to measure the apparent viscosity of the suspension at equilibrium at a given temperature to establish suspension reproducibility

f) Density :

- Specific gravity or density of the suspension is an important parameter.
- A decrease in density often indicates the presence of entrapped air within the structure of the suspension.

Method: Density measurements at a given temperature should be made using well-mixed, uniform suspensions; precision hydrometers facilitate such measurements.

- It is determined by using pycnometer or density bottle.
- Density (D) =Mass/Volume

g) Particle Size Measurement:

- Recently with respect to the importance of particle size distribution in terms of particle characterization and product physical stability testing, Method:-
- 1) Light-Scattering methods for particle detection called photon correlation spectroscopy (PCS).
- (2) By using single particle optical sensing (SPOS)
- (3) With the help of laser diffraction (LD)
- (4) Also by the ultrasound attenuation (UA)

h) Extent of sedimentation:

- It is quantitatively expressed by 2 parameters:

- ➡ Sedimentation volume,
- ➡ Degree of flocculation
- ➡ Sedimentation volume:
- ➡ $F = VU / VO$ = ultimate volume of sediment / initial volume of suspension
- ➡ Where F is sedimentation volume , F' can assume a value of '1', when there is no sedimentation (VU =VO) ,
- ➡ 'F' can also assume a value of 'zero', when sedimentation is complete (VU = 0) ,
- ➡ 'F' value lies between the limits 0 and 1, In general higher the sedimentation volume better is physical stability , A series of suspensions can be prepared using different suspending agents or varying concentrations of same suspending agent.
- ➡ These formulations are transferred into 100 ml measuring cylinders.
- ➡ At different time intervals, sedimentation level in ml is measured.
- ➡ A plot is drawn by taking time on x-axis and VU/VO on y-axis.
- ➡ At zero time, this ratio is equal to one as VU/VO. As the time elapses, sedimentation levels decrease.

DEGREE OF FLOCCULATION:

- ➡ It is defined as $\beta = F/F\alpha$
- ➡ Sedimentation volume of flocculated system = Sedimentation volume of deflocculated system
- ➡ $\beta = VU/V\alpha$
- ➡ Ultimate sedimentation volume of flocculated system -VU

- Ultimate sedimentation volume of deflocculated system -Vα

- If F = Fα, then β will be one.

- If β value is nearer to one, then suspension does not represent flocculated suspension. It indicates it is deflocculated suspension.

- Higher the value of β, greater the physical stability

i) Re dispersibility:

- Re dispersibility can be estimated by shaking the suspension with hands or by

    some mechanical device which is stimulated with motion of human arm.

- Suspension is placed in 100ml graduated cylinder.

- After storage and sedimentation, cylinder is rotated through 360° at 20 rpm. ➡ The end point is taken when base of cylinder is clear of sediment.

- The time required / no of revolutions is noted.

- The shorter the time/ lower the no of revolutions, greater or faster redispersibility

j) Determination of zeta potential :

- This can be determined by using 'zeta meter' which determines by measuring electrophoretic mobility of particles in suspension

- $Z = 4\pi nv/Ee$

- Where, n = viscosity of suspension

- E = applied electric field

- e = dielectrical constant

- V = velocity of particle

- Emulsion:

➥ QC test for Emulsion:

a) Appearance:

➥ The appearance or the emulsion is noted and determined the uniformity of emulsion.

➥ The appearance is noted in transparent glass container

b) Color, odor and taste method:

➥ These characteristics are especially for orally administered emulsion. Variation in color indicates the poor distribution in particle size.

c) Miscibility emulsion: An emulsion will only mix with a liquid that is miscible with its continuous phase therefore an o/w type emulsions miscible with water a w/o emulsion with an oil

➥ Staining evaluation method:

➥ For evaluation of emulsion the staining test is performed.

➥ A dry filter paper impregnated with cobalt chloride turns from blue to pink on exposure to stable o/w emulsion .

➥ Limit: May fail if emulsion is unstable and breaks in presence of electrolyte

➥ Dye Test: Method:

➥ Oil –soluble dye is used. O/w emulsions are pales in color than w/o emulsion and vice versa.

- If examined microscopically, an o/w emulsion will appears as colored globules on a colorless background while aw/o emulsion will appear as colorless globules against a colored background
- Limit: May fail if ionic emulsifier are present

d) Determination of zeta potential: This can be determined by using 'zeta meter' which determines by measuring electrophoretic mobility of particles in suspension.

- $Z = 4\pi nv/Ee$
- Where, n = viscosity of suspension
- E = applied electric field
- e = dielectrical constant
- V = velocity of particle

e) Determination of globule size:

- Size of globule is increased over long storage period i.e. it causes coalescence.
- So to prevent it, globule size should be small.

Globule size is determined by:-

- a) Coulter counter method: in this method, particle diameter is measured and

    also frequency (no of globules per ml) is determined.
- b) Microscopic method: in this method, diameter of globule is measured under a microscope.

➡ c) Laser diffraction sizing method: Size of globule is determined using laser diffraction.

➡ f) Rheological method: This method ensures flow property of emulsion so as to ensure its stability.

➡ Low viscosity of emulsions causes increase in rate of creaming leading to instability. Determination of viscosity is done by using brook field viscometer. A graphical plot of viscosity against time on a log-log scale indicates a linear relationship. This leads to an estimation that viscosity changes with time.

CHAPTER 6

Preparation and Evaluation of Hair and Skin Cosmetics:

Lipstick

Objectives:

1. To discuss hair and skin cosmetics formulations.

2. To formulate and evaluate lipstick and shampoo formulation.

Introduction

- Cosmetic is a Greek word which means to 'adorn' (addition of something decorative to a person or a thing).

- Definition:

- In general, cosmetics are external preparations which are applied on the external parts the body. Cosmetic substances help in improving or changing the outward show of the body and also masks the odour of the body. It protects the skin and keeps it in good condition.

- It may be defined as a substance which comes in contact with various parts of the human body like skin, hair, nail, lips, teeth, and mucous membranes etc.

- Even in earlier days, men and women used to decorate their bodies for improvement of appearance.

- Men used leaves of vegetables and parts of animals whereas women use to wear colored stones and flowers round their neck and wrist.

- Gradually, they start using colored earth and ointments on their face and body.

- Even bangles and necklace made of baked earth materials became very common among the people.

- Eye shadow were made of copper (colored earth) ore and lamp black (colored earth) while red color was used for dyeing of hair.

- Now days, cosmetics are considered as essential components in life.

- They not only, attract the people towards it but also impart psychological effects.

- It has gained popularity in the last 3-4 decades and its use has been increased exponentially both-in males and females.

- The most popular cosmetics are hair dyes, powders and creams.

Examples of Cosmetics

- Skin-care creams

- Powders

- Lotions

- Lipsticks

- Nail polishes

- Eye and face makeup

- Deodorants

- Baby products

- Hair colorants and sprays etc.

Uses

1. They are used as a cleansing, moisturizing and beautifying agent.

2. They help in enhancing attractiveness of the body.

3. They help in altering the appearance of the body without affecting its functions.

4. Sunscreen products help in protecting the body from UV rays and treating sunburns.

5. Acne, wrinkles, dark circles under eyes and other skin imperfections are treated or repaired by treatment products.

6. Cosmetics help in treating skin infection.

Classification

Cosmetics are broadly categorized into four types:

1. Skin Cosmetics

2. Hair Cosmetics

3. Nail Cosmetics

4. Cosmetics for hygiene purpose

Lipsticks

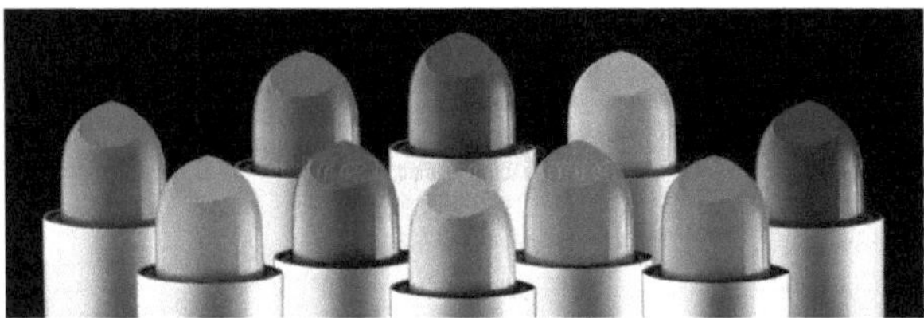

Definition:

- Lipstick may be basically defined as <u>dispersion of the coloring matter in a base consisting of a suitable blend of oils, fats and waxes with suitable perfumes and flavors moulded in the form of sticks to impart attractive gloss and color, when applied on lips.</u>

- Lipsticks provide moist appearance to the lips accentuating them and disguising their defects.

ADVANTAGES OF LIPSTICK

- 1. Beautification effect: no matter what style of lip color you prefer for sharp, bold and dramatic colors, or more natural and subdued shades that can be translucent, it will instantly feel more beautiful.

- 2. Hydration effect: even though some older brands of lipsticks use ingredients that can intake moisture from lips, most of them are very conscientious about hydration and are made to preserve the natural state of our lips. New brands of lipstick can often contain some form of moisturizing additive, such as vitamin E.

- 3. Sunscreen protection effect :it is important and that most people leave their sensitive lips. they are conscious about protecting the rest of the face. Lipstick manufacturers then added sun protection ingredients to their products, enabling to protect lips from external environment and aging effects.

- 4. Posture effect with long and steady tradition of standing in front of the mirror and keeping your posture and body shape in healthy conditions women in the high ages have significantly less problems with their posture and balance.

DISADVANTAGES OF LIPSTICK

- 1. Heavy Metals Studies have shown that lipsticks have concerning levels of chromium, cadmium and magnesium.

- This will result in increasing risk to dangerous diseases and organ damage. High levels of cadmium can be stored in the kidney and finally result in renal failure.

- 2. Lead has been revealed that most of the lipsticks have a dangerously high amount of lead.

- Lead is a neurotoxin and can affect the nervous system. It can also cause brain damage. This is one of the reasons for hormone imbalance and infertility. Even if it's taken in small quantities, it can have drastic effects on the body.

- 3. Formaldehyde and Mineral Oil Formaldehyde is a preservative, which is also known as human carcinogen. Wheezing, coughing, irritation of the eyes and skin are other effects of formaldehyde. Mineral oil is another ingredient which is used in lipstick to block the pores. Many of the harmful effects of lipsticks are due to these chemicals.

- 4. Parabens and Bismuth oxychloride are two ingredients that are used in the manufacturing of lipsticks.

- The harmful effect of lipsticks is due to the carcinogenic property of these two ingredients. The parabens act as preservatives just like the formaldehyde

IDEAL CHARACTERISTICS OF LIPSTICK

1. It should non-toxic.

2. It should be stable both physically and chemically.

3. It should not dry on storage.

4. It should be free from greatly particle.

5. It should maintain lip color for longer period after its application.

6. It should give shiny and smooth appearance free from sweating.

7. It should have pleasant taste, odour and flavor.

8. It should not melt or harden within reasonable variation of climatic temperature.

9. It should be non – irritant.

10. It should have required plasticity.

ANATOMY OF LIPS

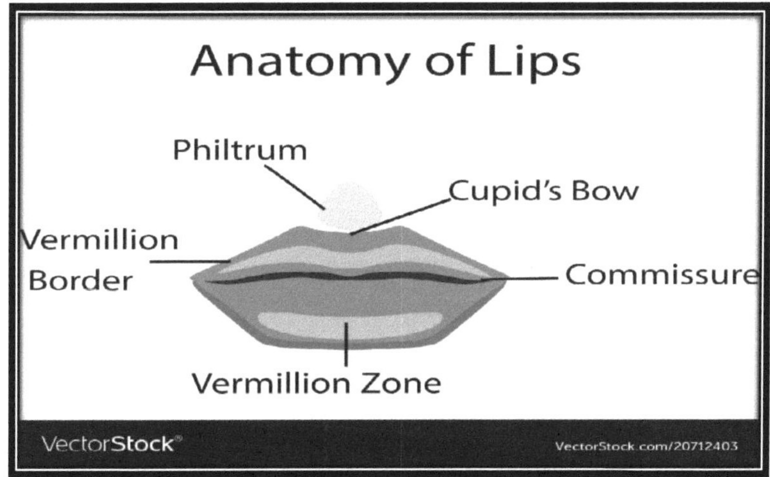

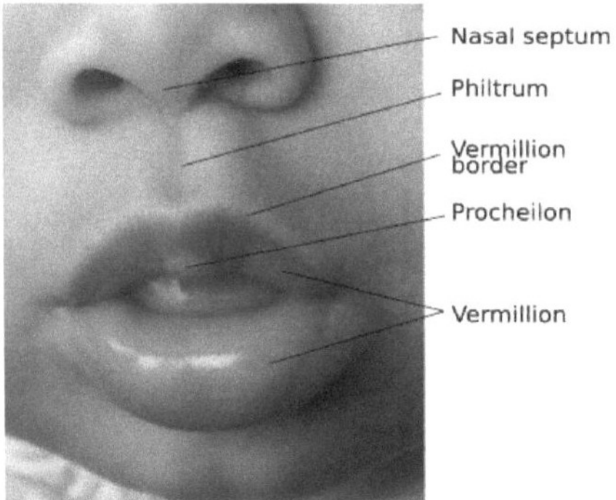

- The anatomy of lips includes upper and lower lips are referred to as the Labium superiusoris and Labium inferiusoris, respectively.

- The junction where the lips meet the surrounding skin of the mouth area is the vermilion border, and the typically reddish area within the borders is called the vermilion zone.

- The vermilion border of the upper lip is known as the Cupid's bow..

- The vertical groove extending from the procheilon to the nasal septum is called the philtrum.

- The skin of the lip, with three to five cellular layers, is very thin compared to typical face skin, which has up to 16 layers. With light skin color, the lip skin contains fewer melanocytes (cells which produce melanin pigment, which give skin its color).

- Because of this, the blood vessels appear through the skin of the lips, which leads to their notable red coloring. With darker skin color this effect is less prominent, as in this case the skin of the lips contains more melanin and thus is visually darker.

Formulation of lipsticks

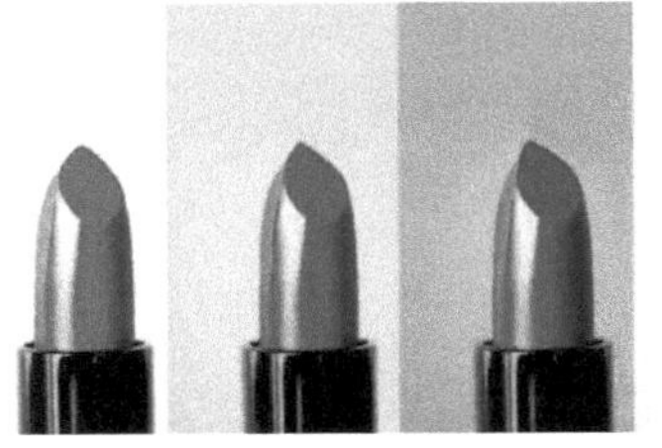

The lipstick base is made by mixing the oils and waxes in varying proportions in order to obtain a desirable viscosity and melting point.

The solid components of the formulation are mostly natural waxes which may be classified as follows:

a. The hydrocarbon waxes: Example: White bees wax

b. The mineral waxes: Example: Ozokerite, ceresine

c. Hard waxes: Example: Carnauba wax, candelilla wax, hard paraffin etc.

a. Micro crystalline waxes

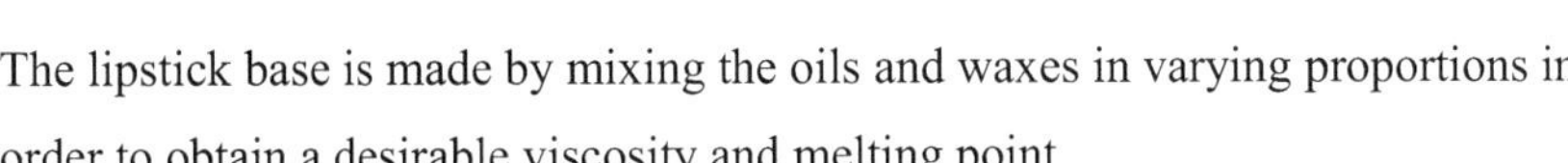

The solid components / waxes | White bees wax

(a) The hydrocarbon waxes — White bees wax

(b) The mineral waxes — Ozokerite wax, ceresine wax

(c) Hard waxes — Carnauba wax, candelilla wax, hard paraffin

(d) Micro crystalline waxes

The liquid components	Mineral oils, vegetable oils, castor oils, butyl stearate, Glycol, water, silicon-fluids, IPM (isopropyl maleate)
The softening components	Anhydrous lanoline, lanolin cocoa butter, lecithin, petrolatum
The coloring agents	Carmine (source :**the shells of the cochineal beetle**), dyestuff stain, pigmented stain.

Ingredients	Example
Pearlescent pigments	Guanine crystals, bismuth oxychloride
Opacifying agents	Titanium dioxide
Perfumeries	Rose oil,, cinnamon oil, lavender oil etc.
Miscellaneous agents :	Parabens
(a) Preservatives	BHA (**beta-hydroxy acid**), BHT(butylated hydroxytoluene),
(b) Antioxidants	
(c) Flavouring agents	tocopherol etc.

Cinnamon oil, spearmint oil etc.

Evaluation of Lipsticks

The evaluation studies are important in order to determine the efficiency, stability and the consistency of the finished product.

EVALUATION PARAMETERS OF LIPSTICK

1. Melting point: -The determination of melting point is done in order to determine the storage characteristics of the product.

The inciting point of lipstick base should be between 60 to 65°C in order to avoid the sensation of friction or dryness during application.

The method of determination is known as capillary tube method:

The evaluation studies are important in order to determine the efficiency, stability and the consistency of the finished product.

EVALUATION PARAMETERS OF LIPSTICK

1. Melting point: -The determination of melting point is done in order to determine the storage characteristics of the product.

The inciting point of lipstick base should be between 60 to 65°C in order to avoid the sensation of friction or dryness during application.

The method of determination is known as capillary tube method:

EVALUATION PARAMETERS OF LIPSTICK: Melting point

a) In this method, about 50 mg of lipstick is taken and is inserted into a glass capillary tube open at both ends.

(b) The capillary tube is ice cooled for about hrs. and then placed in a beaker containing

hot water and a magnetic stirrer.

(c) The temperature at which material starts moving through the capillary is said to be

the melting point temperature.

(d) Another important parameter is the droop point which determines the temperature at

which the product starts oozing out the oil and becomes flattened out.

(e) The melting point should be higher than the droop point which determines the safe

handling and storage of finished product.

2- Breaking Load Point Test:

This test is done in order to determine the strength and hardness of the lipstick.

In this method, the lipstick is placed horizontal position I inch from the base and weights with increasing loads are attached to it.

The weight at which the lipstick starts breaking, known as the breaking load point.

The test shall be carried out in specific condition and at about 25 ° C temperatures.

3- Determination of thixotropic character:

- This is a test for determining the uniformity in viscosity of base.

- The instrument used for the determination of thixotropic character is known as the penetrometer.

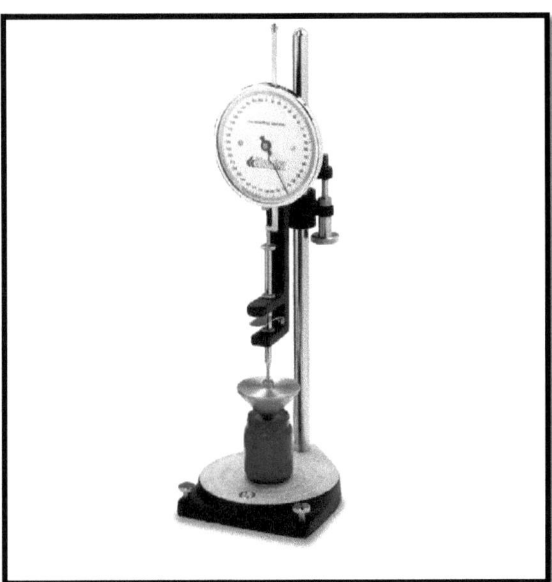

4- Microbiological tests:

- The test is carried out in order to determine the extent of contamination either from the raw materials or mould.

- The test involves the plating of known mass of sample on two different culture media for the growth of microorganism and incubating them for a specific period of time.

- The extent of contamination can be estimated by counting the number of colonies.

5- Test for rancidity:

- The oxidation of oil such as castor oil and many other ingredients may result in bad odour and taste and also result in a sticky product.

- The test for rancidity can be done by using hydrogen peroxide and determining its peroxide number.

6- Test for the Application Force:

- This is a test to determine the force to be applied during application.

- In this method, two lipsticks are cut to obtain flat surfaces which are placed one above other.

- A smooth paper is placed between them which is attached to a dynamometer to determine force required to pull the paper indicates the force application.

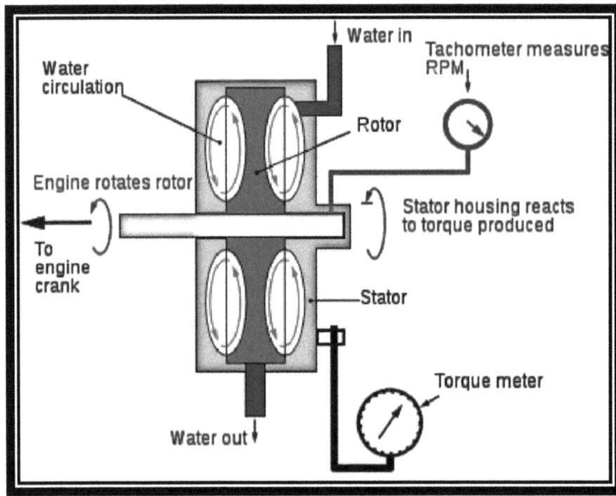

7- Storage Stability:

- This test is done in order to determine the stability of product during storage.

8- Stability to Oxidation:

- The oxidation characteristics of the finished product are determined in order to check the stability of the product to oxidation.

- The extent of oxidation can be determined by peroxide number of product after exposure or substance to oxygen for a specific period of time.

- 9- Determination of Surface Characteristics:

- The study of surface property of the product is carried out in order to check the formation crystal on the surface or the contamination by microorganism or formation of wrinkles and the exudation of liquid.

- 10- Determination of Colour dispersion:

- The test is done in order to determine the uniform dispersion of color particle.

- The size of the particle is determined by the microscopic studies and it should not be more than 50µ.

DEFECTS IN LIPSTICK

1. Sweating: - It is the most common problem of lipstick formulation due to high oil content or inferior oil binding. It may rise in any climate or temperature range.

2. Bleeding: - This refers separation of colored to the liquids from the waxy base.

3. Streaking: - A thin line or band of a different color or substances appears on the finished product.

Molding Related Problems

4. Laddering: -Lipstick does not look smooth or homogenous after congealing and setting but instead has a multilayered appearance.

5. Deformation: -This is a molding problem where the shape of the lipstick looks deformed .It is noticeable and appears on both sides of the lipstick.

6. Cratering: -This appears in split molding and it shows up flaming when stick develops dimples.

7. Mushy Failure: - This is a problem in which the central core of the lipstick lacks structure and breaks

OUTCOME

- This chapter covers the general information about cosmetics and lipstick preparation, advantages, disadvantages, evaluation and defects.

CHAPTER 7

Preparation and Evaluation of Hair and Skin Cosmetics:
Shampoo

Objectives:

1. To discuss hair and skin cosmetics formulations.
2. To formulate and evaluate shampoo formulation.

Objectives

- 1. Introduction

- 2. Types of Shampoos
- 3. Product Ingredients
- 4. Formulation
- 5. Evaluation of Shampoos

Introduction

Definition:

A shampoo is a preparation of a surfactant (i.e. surface active material) in a suitable form – liquid, solid or powder – which when used under the specified conditions will remove surface grease, dirt, and skin debris from the hair shaft and scalp without adversely affecting the user.

Requirements of a Shampoo

1. It should effectively and completely remove dust or soil, excessive sebum or other fatty substances and loose corneal cells from the hair.

2. It should produce a good amount of foam to satisfy the psychological requirements of the user.

3.   It should be easily removed on rinsing with water.

4. It should leave the hair non-dry, soft, lustrous with good manageability and minimum fly away.

5. It should impart a pleasant fragrance to the hair.

6. It should not cause any side-effects / irritation to skin or eye.

7. It should not make the hand rough and chapped

Types of Shampoo

- ➢ Powder Shampoo
- ➢ Liquid Shampoo
- ➢ Lotion Shampoo
- ➢ Cream Shampoo
- ➢ Jelly Shampoo
- ➢ Aerosol Shampoo
- ➢ Specialized Shampoo
    - • • Conditioning Shampoo
    - • • Anti- dandruff Shampoo

ANIONIC SURFACTANTS		
CLASS	EXAMPLE	COMMENT
Alkyl benzene sulfonates	Sodium dodecyl benzene sulfonate	Tend to yield an "airy" or low density foam and often are drying to the hair
Primary alkyl sulfates	Lauric acid, stearic acid and their salts	Good lathering effect in hard water, free from rancidity, easy to wash.
Secondary alcohol sulfates	Sodium sec-lauryl sulfate	Low cost, dispersing and emulsifying action, dissapointing as detergets and shampoo components

- • • Two Layer Shampoo

Alkyl benzene polyoxyethylene sulfonates	Triton X200	Stable in acid or alkaline solution, excellent emulsifier, detergent and wetting agent; extremely stable at pH of skin
Sulfated monoglycerides	Lauric monoglyceride ammonium sulfate	Stable in hard water
Alkyl ether sulfates	Derivatives of lauryl alcohol ether with PEG	Good cleansers, act as solvents for non polar additives
Sarcosines	Lauroyl and cocoyl sarcosines	Excellent foaming and conditioning action
Sulfosuccinates	Aerosol OT	Less irritating to skin and eye (baby shampoo)
Maypon	Protalbinic and lysalbinic acid derivatives (maypon 4C)	Hydrolysation product of proteins with fatty acid chlorides in presence of alkali

CLASS	EXAMPLE	COMMENTS
Fatty acid alkanolamides (should not be used > 15%)	Lauric monoethanolamide	Improves solubility of SLS
	Stearic ethanolamide	Pearlescent thickener
	Oleic ethanolamides	Hair conditioning agents
Polyalkoxylated derivatives	Ethoxylated fatty alcohols	Stable in wide range of pH; stabilizing emulsifying and opacifying properties

	Block polymers (pluronics)	Good rinsability, can be used in high %
	Sorbitol esters (TWEENS)	Solubilizers and emulsifiers, used in baby shampoos
Amine oxides	Coconut and dodecyl dimethyl amine oxides	Foam booster and anti-static agents
AMPHOTERIC SURFACTANTS		
N-alkyl aminoacids	β – aminoacid derivatives	Foaming agents
	Aspargine derivatives	Compatible with both anionic and cationic surfactants
Betains	Amido betains	High foaming properties, mild.
Alkyl imidazoline	MIRANOL^{TM}	Baby shampoos

PRODUCT INGREDIENTS

- Surfactants are the main component of shampoo. Mainly anionic surfactants are used.
- The raw materials used in the manufacture of shampoos are:
- 1. Principal surfactants: Provide detergency and foam.
- 2. Secondary surfactants: Improve detergency, foam and hair condition.
- 3. Other additives.

CLEANSING ACTION OF SHAMPOO

- A surfactant consists of two part- one hydrophilic (water loving) while the other is hydrophobic in nature.

Surfactants

- Anionic surfactants are mostly used (good foaming properties). The hydrophilic portion carries a negative charge which results in superior foaming, cleaning and end result attributes.
- Non-ionic surfactants have good cleansing properties but do not have sufficient foaming power.
- Cationic surfactants are toxic and are hence not used. However, they may be used in low concentration in hair conditioners.
- Ampholytics, being expensive, are generally not used. However, they are mainly used as secondary surfactants and good hair conditioners.

ADDITIVES

Conditioning agents: Lanolin, mineral oil, herbal extracts, egg derivatives.

- **Foam builders**: Lauryl monoethanolamide, sarcosinates
- **Viscosity modifiers** :
    - Electrolytes – NH_4Cl, $NaCl$
    - Natural gums – Gum Karaya, tragacanth, alginates
    - Cellulose derivatives – Hydroxy ethyl cellulose, methyl cellulose
    - Carboxy vinyl polymers – Carbopol 934
    - Others – PVP, Phosphate esters.
- **Sequestering agents** : EDTA
- **Opacifying agents** : Alkanol amides of higher fatty acids, Propylene glycol, Mg Ca and Zn salts of stearic acid, spermaceti, etc.
- **Clarifying agents** :
    - Solubilizing alcohols – ethanol, isopropanol

- Phosphates –
- Non-ionic solubilizers – polyethoxyated alcohols and esters.

ADDITIVES

- **Perfumes** : Herbal, fruity or floral fragrances.
- **Preservatives** : Methyl and propyl paraben, formaldehyde (most effective).
- **Anti-dandruff agents**: The shampoos contain small amount of these actives, which are in contact with the scalp for only a short time. In order to be effective the active ingredient must work in the oil- water environment of the scalp and must be readily substantive to the scalp for continuing activity.
- Ex: Selenium sulfide, zinc pyrithione, salicylic acid.

POWDER SHAMPOO	
Henna powder	5%
Soap powder	50%
Sodium carbonate	22.5%
Potassium carbonate	7.5%
Borax	15%
Perfume	q.S

LOTION SHAMPOO	
TLS(Triethanolamine Lauryl Sulfate TLS)	35%
Glyceryl monostearate	2%
Magnesium stearate	1%
Water	Upto 100%
Color	q.s
Perfume, preservatives	q.s

LIQUID SHAMPOO	
SLS	40%
NaCl (to desired viscosity)	2-4%
Water	Upto 100%
Perfume, color, preservatives	q.s

FORMULATIONS

CREAM SHAMPOO	
SLS	38%
Cetyl alcohol	7%

Water	Upto 100%
Color, perfume	q.S
Preservative	q.s

AEROSOL SHAMPOO

TLS	60%
Coconut diethanolamide	2%
Water	Upto 90%
Propellent	10%
Color, perfume, preservative	q,.s

JELLY SHAMPOOS

Alkyl dimethyl benzalkonium chloride	15%
TLS (40%)	28%
Coconut ditethanolamide	7%
HPMC	1%
Water	Upto 100%
Color, perfume, preservative	q.s

CONDITIONING SHAMPOOS

Steryl dimethyl benzyl ammonium chloride	5.5%
Ethylene glycol monostearate	2%
Cetyl alcohol	2.5%
Water	Upto 100%
Color, perfume, preservative	q.s

TWO LAYER SHAMPOO

SLS (**Sodium Lauryl Sulphate**)	27%
Cocamidopropylamine oxide	5%
Lauramine DEA(mixture of ethanolamides of lauric acid)	1%
Lactic acid (50%)	1%
Formaldehyde	0.1%

BABY SHAMPOO

Magnesium lauryl sulfate (27.5%)	11%
Cocamidopropyl betaine (30%)	5%
Polysorbate 20	1%
PEG 600	3.5%
Perfume	q.S
Preservative	q.S
Citric acid	To pH 6
Color	q.S
Water (deionised); Aqua (INCI)	To 100%

FORMULATIONS

ANTI-DANDRUFF SHAMPOO	
Thymol	0.05%
Menthol	0.1%
Camphor	0.1%
TLS	55%
Water	upto 100
Color, perfume, preservative	q.s

ANTI-DANDRUFF SHAMPOO	
Selenium sulfide	2.5%
Bentonite	5%
SLS paste	35%
Water	upto 100
Color, perfume, preservative	q.s

HERBAL SHAMPOO	
Natural essential oil blend	0.5%
Cyamopsis tetragonoloba (Guar Gum)	1%
Camellia sinensis (Green Tea) extract	2%
Glycerin	1%
Hydrolysed wheat protein	2.5%
Salvia officinalis (Sage) leaf extract	1.5%
Salvia officinalis	1.5%
Glyceryl oleate	1%
Polysorbate 20	0.5%

Potassium sorbate	5%
Aloe barbadensis (Aloe vera) extract	0.5%
Arctium minus (Burdock) root extract	0.5%
Disodium coco-glucoside sulfosuccinate	0.5%
Preservatives	q.s.
Water	Upto 100%

Salvia officinalis

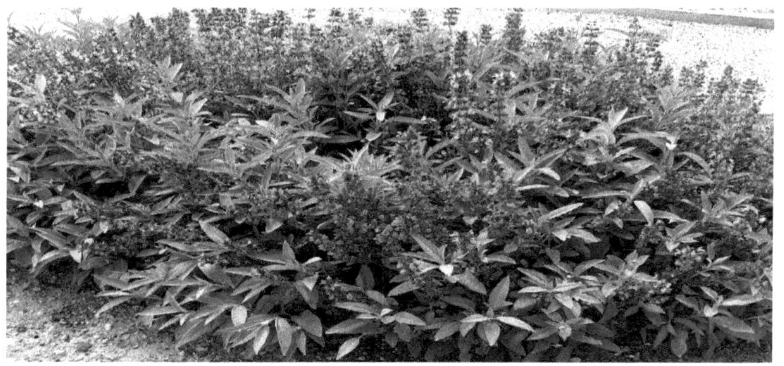

Arctium minus

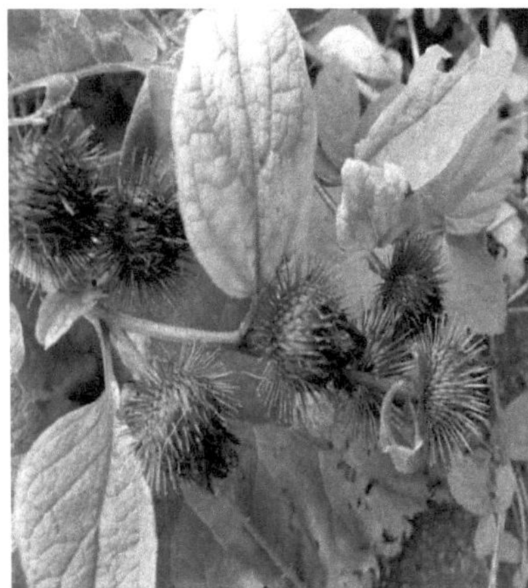 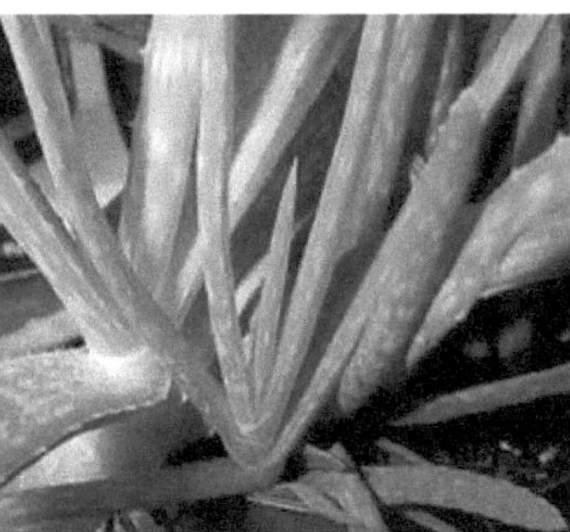

Evaluation of Shampoos

Performance characteristics

1) Foam and foam stability

2) Detergency and cleaning action

3) Effect of water hardness

4) Surface Tension and wetting

5) Surfactant content and analysis

6) Rinsing

7) Conditioning action

8) Softness

9) Luster

10)   Lubricity

11)   Body, texture and set retention

12)   Irritation and toxicity

13)   Dandruff control

14)   Microbiological assay

15)   Eye irritancy test

Product characteristics

1) Fragnance
2) Consistency
3) Package

1. Foam and foam stability:

• The Ross-Miles foam column test is accepted. 200 ml of surfactant solution is dropped into a glass column containing 50ml of the same solution. The height of the foam generated is measured immediately and again after a specified time interval, and is considered proportional to the volume.

• Barnett and Powers developed a latherometer to measure the effect of variables such as water hardness, type of soil and quantity of soil on foam speed, volume and stability.

• Fredell and Read titrated actual standard oiled heads of hair with additive increments of shampoo until a persistent lather end point appeared.

1. Foam and foam stability:

- The Ross-Miles foam column test is accepted.
- 200 ml of surfactant solution is dropped into a glass column containing 50ml of the same solution.
- The height of the foam generated is measured immediately and again after a specified time interval, and is considered proportional to the volume.
- Barnett and Powers developed a lather meter to measure the effect of variables such as water hardness, type of soil and quantity of soil on foam speed, volume and stability.

- Fredell and Read titrated actual standard oiled heads of hair with additive increments of shampoo until a persistent lather end point appeared.

2. Detergency and cleaning action:

- Cleansing power is evaluated by the method of Barnet and Powers
- 5gm sample of soiled human hair is placed at 35°c in 200 ml of water containing of 1 gm of shampoo.
- The flask is shaken 50 times a minute for 4 minutes. Then washed once again with sufficient amount of water, then after filter the hair dried and weighed.
- The amount of soil is removed under these condition is calculated.

3. Wetting Action:

- Canvas disk sinking test:
- 6 canvas disk made up of mount veron cotton 1 inch in diameter is floated on the surface of the solution, and the time required to sink is measured accurately.

4.Microbiological assay::

- staphylococcus   aureus   (ATCC6532)
- The wells are dig on agar plates with sterilised well digger aseptically.
- •Take 100μml of each sample, add to well aseptically.
- Incubate the plates at 37°C for 24 hrs to 48 hrs.
- Observe the effectiveness of sample on culture growing on the agar plate and we can see the effectiveness of sample in the form of zone of inhibition around each well containing different sample.

<u>**5. Evaluation of eye irritancy:**</u>

- The test calls for dropping 0.1 ml of liquid shampoo in the conjunctiva sac of one eye of the rabbit, the other eye serving as control.
- •   In the case of the first three animals, the treated eye remains unwashed. Since washing the eye may or may not alleviate symptoms of injury.
- The six remaining animals are divided into two equal groups.
- •   In the first of these groups eyes instilled with the substances are washed with 20 ml of lukewarm water two seconds after treatment and in the second group after instillation.
- •   Readings are then made at 24, 48 and 72 hr and again four and seven days after treatment.
- •   If the lesions have not cleared up in seven days the test material is considered as severe irritant.

8. Viscosity:

- Viscosity of the liquid shampoo is determined using a Brookefield viscometer
- 100 mL of the shampoo is taken in a beaker and the spindle is dipped in it for about 5 min and then the reading is taken.

Expected learning outcomes

The students may be able to develop the formulation and evaluation of different types of shampoo.

CHAPTER 8

Quality control of vaccines

A Quick Glimpse…

- Active vs. Passive Immunization

- Designing Vaccines

- Diphtheria and Tetanus Vaccine

- Bacillus Calmette-Guérin Vaccine (BCG)

INTRODUCTION

Immunity

- Ability of human body to tolerate the presence of material indigenous to the body and to eliminate foreign material

- This discriminatory ability provide protection from infectious disease

- Indicated by the presence of antibody to the organism causing infectious disease

IMMUNITY
INNATE
ADAPTIVE
1. ANATOMICAL BARRIER
2. PHYSIOLOGICAL BARRIER
3. PHAGOCYTIC BARRIER
4. INFLAMMATORY BARRIER
ACTIVE
PASSIVE
NATURAL IMMUNITY
ARTIFICIAL IMMUNITY
NATURAL IMMUNITY
ARTIFICIAL IMMUNITY
Active immunity
Passive immunity
Mumps 12/9/79
Naturally acquired
Naturally acquired
Artificially acquired
Artificially acquired
SERUM

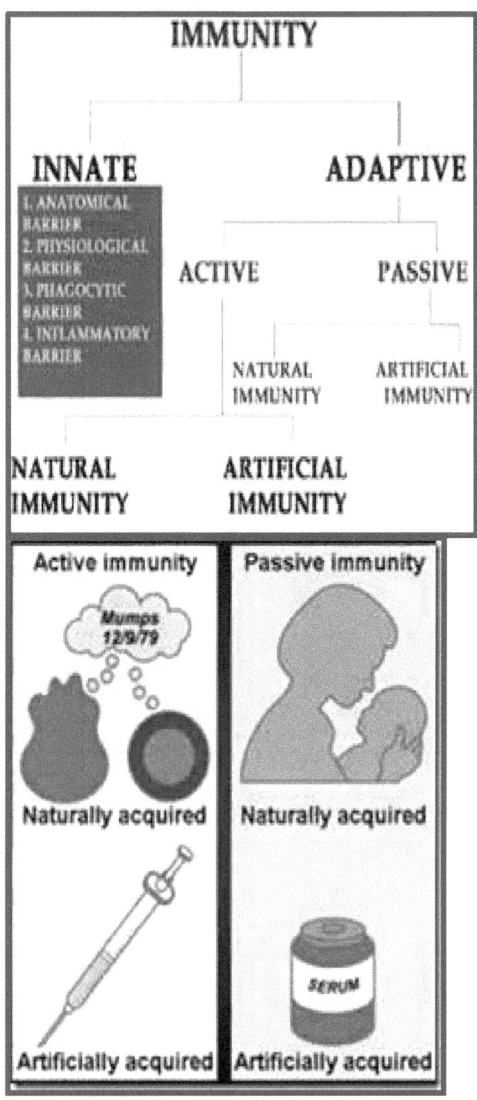

Vaccines

Vaccines are whole or parts of microorganisms administered to prevent an infectious disease

Two Types of Immunization

- Passive Immunization

    - Methods of acquisition include natural maternal antibodies, antitoxins, and immune globulins

    - Protection transferred from another person or animal

    - Active Immunization

    - Methods of acquisition include natural infection, vaccines (many types), and toxoids

    - Relatively permanent

ACQUISITION OF PASSIVE AND ACTIVE IMMUNITY

Type	Acquired through
Passive immunity	Natural maternal antibody
	Immune globulin[*]
	Antitoxin[†]
Active immunity	Natural infection
	Vaccines[‡]
	Attenuated organisms
	Inactivated organisms
	Purified microbial macromolecules
	Cloned microbial antigens
	(alone or in vectors)
	Multivalent complexes
	Toxoid[§]

Passive Immunization

- Can occur naturally via transfer of maternal antibodies across placenta to fetus

- Injection with preformed antibodies

    - Human or animal antibodies can be used

    - Injection of animal Ab's prevalent before vaccines

- Effects are only temporary

Conditions Warranting Passive Immunization

1. Deficiency in synthesis of Ab as a result of congenital or acquired B-cell defects

2. Susceptible person is exposed to a disease that will cause immediate complications (time is the biggest issue)

3. Disease is already present

Common Agents For Passive Immunization

COMMON AGENTS USED FOR PASSIVE IMMUNIZATION	
Disease	Agent
Black widow spider bite	Horse antivenin
Botulism	Horse antitoxin
Diphtheria	Horse antitoxin
Hepatitis A and B	Pooled human immune gamma globulin
Measles	Pooled human immune gamma globulin
Rabies	Pooled human immune gamma globulin
Snake bite	Horse antivenin
Tetanus	Pooled human immune gamma globulin or horse antitoxin

The Immune System and Passive Immunization

- The transfer of antibodies will not trigger the immune system

- There is NO presence of memory cells

- Risks are included

    - Recognition of the immunoglobulin epitope by self immunoglobluin paratopes

    - Some individuals produce IgE molecules specific for passive antibody, leading to mast cell degranulation

- Some individuals produce IgG or IgM molecules specific for passive antibody, leading to hypersensitive reactions

Active Immunization

- Natural Infection with microorganism or artificial acquisition (vaccine)

- Both stimulate the proliferation of T and B cells, resulting in the formation of effector and **memory** cells

- The formation of memory cells is the basis for the relatively permanent effects of vaccinations

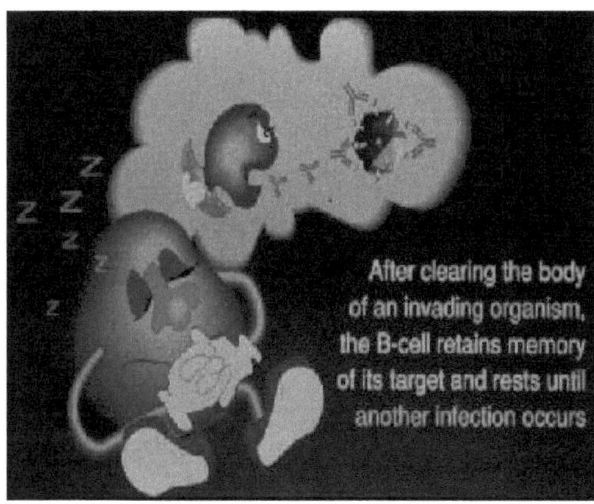

Principles Underlying Vaccination

- Concept of Immunity

    - Self vs. Non-self

    - Antigen specificity

    - Indicated by presence of effector cells

Vaccinations

RECOMMENDED CHILDHOOD IMMUNIZATION SCHEDULE IN THE UNITED STATES, JANUARY–DECEMBER 1999

Vaccine*	Birth	1 mo	2 mos	4 mos	6 mos	12 mos	15 mos	18 mos	4–6 yrs
Hepatitis B		+							
			+			+			
Diphtheria, tetanus, pertussis‡			+	+	+		+		+
H. influenzae, type b			+	+	+	+			
Poliovirus§			+	+		+			
Rotavirus¶			+	+	+				
Measles, mumps, rubella						+			+
Varicella‡							+		

Boosters (multiple inoculations) are required

Interference of passive maternal antibodies

Diphtheria and Tetanus Vaccine

DTwP Vaccines

> Compose of diphtheria & tetanus toxoids & killed whole cell pertussis bacilli adsorbed on insoluble aluminium salts (adjuvants)

> Vaccine storage: 2-8°C; Dose: 0.5 ml **deep** i.m.

> Immunity against all three components wanes over the next 6-12 years; therefore regular boosting needed

> Most adverse reactions are due to pertussis component

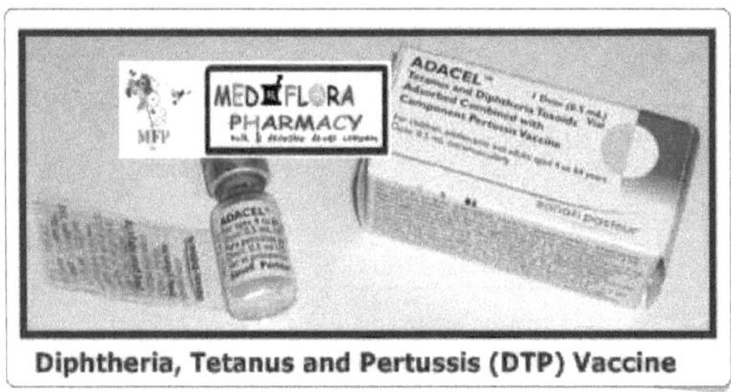

Diphtheria, Tetanus and Pertussis (DTP) Vaccine

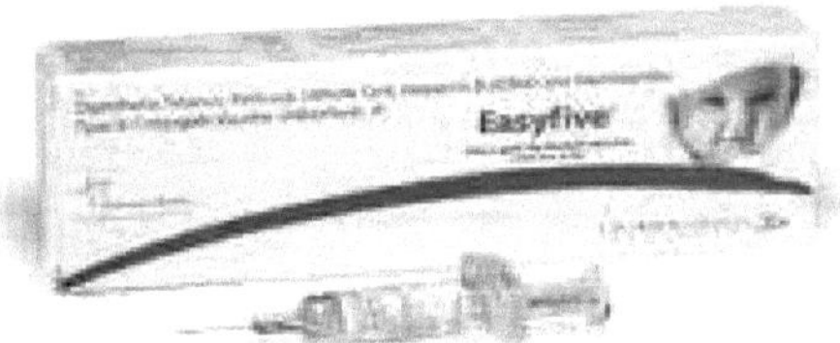

Adsorbed Diphtheria and Tetanus Vaccine

- They are formol toxoids

- Prepared from toxins produced by the growth of *Corynebacterium diphtheriae & Clostridium tetani*, resp., with a mineral adsorbent (hydrated Aluminium. phosphate or Al. hydroxide).

- Isotonic with blood

- Suitable antimicrobial preservatives may be added.

Specific toxicity of the diphtheria and tetanus components :

Comply with the following test:

- - inject SC 5 times the single human dose stated on the label into each of 5 healthy guinea-pigs, (250-350 g), that have not previously been treated with any material that will interfere with the test.

- The vaccine does not comply with the test

- If within 42 days of the injection any of the animals shows signs of or dies from diphtheria toxaemia or tetanus,.

- If more than 1 animal dies from non-specific causes, repeat the test once;

- if more than 1 animal dies in the second test, the vaccine does not comply with the test.

-

IDENTIFICATION;

- Immunochemical method.

- Dissolve in the vaccine to be examined sufficient sodium citrate to give a 100 g/l solution.

- Maintain at 37 °C for about 16 h and centrifuge.

- The clear supernatant liquid reacts with a suitable diphtheria/tetanus antitoxin, giving a precipitate.

TESTS

- Aluminium: Maximum 1.25 mg per single human dose, (if aluminium hydroxide or hydrated aluminium phosphate is used as the adsorbent)

- Free formaldehyde : Maximum 0.2 g/l.

- Antimicrobial preservative; Not less than the minimum amount shown to be effective and is not greater than 115 per cent of the quantity stated on the label.

- Sterility

ASSAY

Diphtheria component: The lower confidence limit (P = 0.95) of the estimated potency is not less than 30 IU per single human dose

Tetanus component

The lower confidence limit (P = 0.95) of the estimated potency is not less

than 40

Bacillus Calmette-Guérin Vaccine (BCG)

IU per single human dose

Preparation of live bacteria derived from a culture of the bacillus of Calmette and Guérin (Mycobacterium bovis BCG) whose capacity to protect against tuberculosis has been established

BCG vaccine shall be produced by

- a staff consisting of healthy persons who do not work with with virulent strains of *Mycobacterium tuberculosis,*

- *nor shall they be exposed to a known risk of tuberculosis infection*

- Staff are examined periodically for tuberculosis

BCG vaccine is susceptible to sunlight

- All cultures and vaccines are protected from

  - direct sunlight and ultraviolet light

- at all stages of manufacture, testing and storage.

IDENTIFICATION: By microscopic examination of the bacilli in stained smears

- acid-fast property and

- by the characteristic appearance of colonies grown on solid medium

TESTS

- Virulent mycobacteria

- Inject SC or IM into each of 6 guinea-pigs (250-400 g) and having received no treatment likely to interfere with the test, a quantity of vaccine equivalent to at least 50 human doses.

- Observe the animals for at least 42 days.

- At the end of this period, euthanise the guinea-pigs and

- examine by autopsy for signs of infection with TB

The vaccine complies with the test

- if none of the guinea-pigs shows signs of TB &

- if not more than 1 animal dies during the observation period.

- If 2 animals die during this period and autopsy does not reveal signs of TB repeat the test on 6 other guinea-pigs.

The vaccine complies with the test

- if not more than 1 animal dies during the 42 days following the injection and autopsy does not reveal any sign of TB.

Excessive dermal reactivity

- Use 6 healthy, white or pale-coloured guinea-pigs (weighing not less than 250 g).

- Inject intradermally into each guinea-pig, according to a randomised plan, 0.1 ml of the reconstituted vaccine and of 2 tenfold serial dilutions of the vaccine and identical doses of the comparison vaccine

- Observe the lesions formed at the site of the injection for 4 weeks.

- The vaccine complies with the test if the reaction it produces is not markedly different from that produced by the comparison vaccine.

- **Water**: Not more than the limit approved for the particular product, determined by a suitable method.

Temperature stability

- Maintain samples of the freeze-dried vaccine at 37 °C for 4 weeks.

- Determine the number of viable units in the heated vaccine and in unheated vaccine

- The number of viable units in the heated vaccine is not less than 20 per cent that in unheated vaccine

Expected learning outcomes

- The students may be able to explain the quality control tests for vaccines

CHAPTER 9

Good Manufacturing Practices (GMP)

Objectives

- Definition

- Main Components

- Principles of GMP

- Standards for CGMP

Definition

- Good Manufacturing Practice is a set of regulations, codes, and guidelines for the manufacture of drug substances and drug products, medical devices, in vivo and in vitro diagnostic products, and foods.

- Overall, it protects both company and consumer from negative food ad drug safety events.

<u>Some areas that can influence the safety and quality of products that GMP guideline and regulation address are the following :</u>

1. Quality management

2. Sanitation and hygiene

3. Building and facilities

4. Equipment

5. Raw materials

6. Personnel

7. Validation and qualification

8. Complaints

9. Documentation and recordkeeping

10.Inspections & quality audits

What is the difference between GMP and cGMP?

- Good Manufacturing Practices (GMP) and current Good Manufacturing Practices (cGMP) are, in most cases, **interchangeable**.

- GMP is the basic regulation promulgated by the US Food and Drug Administration (FDA) under the authority of the Federal Food, Drug, and Cosmetic Act to ensure that manufacturers are taking proactive steps to guarantee their products are safe and effective.

- cGMP, on the other hand, was implemented by the FDA <u>to ensure continuous improvement in the approach of manufacturers to product quality.</u>

- It implies a constant commitment to the <u>highest available quality standards through the use of up-to-date systems and technologies.</u>

What are the 5 Main Components of Good Manufacturing Practice?

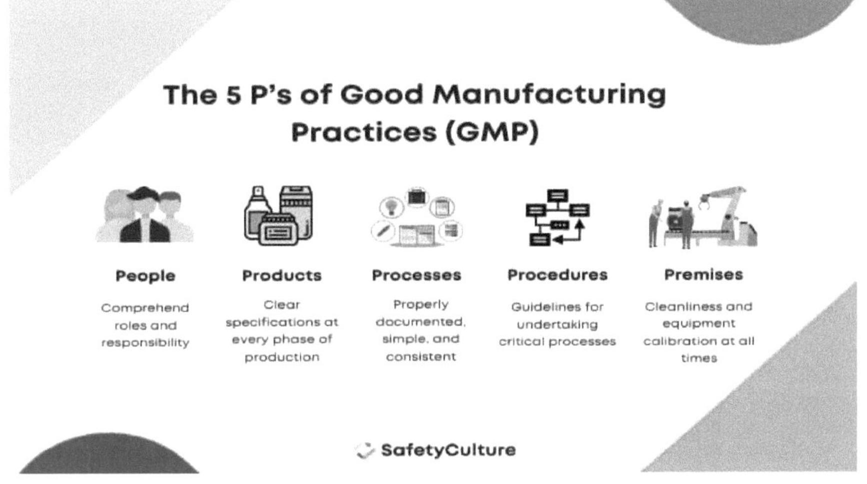

What are the 10 Principles of GMP?

1. Create Standard Operating Procedures (SOPs)

2. Enforce / Implement SOPs and work instructions

3. Document procedures and processes

4. Validate the effectiveness of SOPs

5. Design and use working systems

6. Maintain systems, facilities, and equipment

7. Develop job competence of workers

8. Prevent contamination through cleanliness

9. Prioritize quality and integrate into workflow

10. Conduct <u>GMP audits</u> regularly to uphold GMP standards.

Quality team

Have a team of skilled workers that will focus on improving current manufacturing procedures and complying with GMP.

1. **Validation**

   Validation is the documented act of demonstrating instruments, processes, and activities that are regularly used or done.

2. This is done to check if they function according to expectations. GMP can involve a number of things to be validated, but it's good to focus on the following processes:

   1. Process validation

   2. Cleaning and sanitation validation

   3. Computer system validation

   4. Analytical method validation

3. Surprise Audits

A surprise audit every now and then can help gain a more accurate insight into what goes on in the facility. Identify real root causes of non-compliance and take action before it progresses into a larger issue.

4. Compliance Training

Providing compliance training to staff is the best way to ensure compliance with GMP standards.

- Help staff gain a better understanding of GMP and continually improve operations or systems in place to ensure standards are GMP-compliant.

- All employees should receive training on recordkeeping, sanitation, proper equipment handling, and labeling, and SOPs to minimize errors and maintain compliance.

<u>**Standards for CGMP**</u>

- Regulations established by FDA to ensure that minimum standards are met for drug product quality

- First GMP regulations were promulgated in 1963 under provisions of Kefauver-Harris Drug Amendments

- Since then periodically revised and updated.

- cGMP regulations establish requirements for all aspects of pharmaceutical manufacture.

- Apply to domestic and to foreign suppliers and manufacturers whose bulk components and finished pharmaceutical products are imported, distributed or sold in this country.

- To ensure compliance, FDA inspects facilities and production records of all firms covered by these regulations.

Definitions

- **<u>Active ingredient:</u>** Any component that is intended to furnish pharmacologic activity or other direct effect in diagnosis, cure, mitigation, treatment of disease or to affect the structure or function of the body of man or other animals.

- **<u>Batch:</u>** Specific quantity of drug of uniform specified quality produced according to single manufacturing order during the same cycle of manufacture.

- **<u>Certification</u>**: Documented testimony by qualified authorities that a system qualification, calibration, validation, has been performed appropriately and that the results are acceptable.

- **<u>Drug product</u>**: Finished form that contains an active drug and inactive ingredients. Term may also include a form that does not contain an active ingredient, such as placebo.

- **<u>Inactive ingredient:</u>** Any component other than the active ingredient in a drug product.

- **<u>Master record:</u>** Record containing the formulation, specifications, manufacturing procedures, quality assurance requirements and labeling of a finished product.

- **<u>Quality control:</u>** Regulatory process through which industry measures actual quality performance, compares it with standards and acts on the difference

- **<u>Quality audit:</u>** A documented activity performed in accordance with established procedures on a planned and periodic basis to verify compliance with procedures to ensure quality.

- **<u>Quarantine</u>** : An area that is marked, designated, or set aside for holding of incoming components prior to acceptance, testing and qualification for use.

- **<u>Representative sample:</u>** A sample that accurately portrays the whole.

- **<u>Reprocessing:</u>** The activity whereby the finished product or any of its components is recycled through all or part of the manufacturing process.

- **<u>Strength:</u>** The concentration of the drug substance per unit dose or volume.

- **<u>Validation:</u>** Documented evidence that a system (e.g. equipment, software, controls) does what it purports to do.

- **<u>Process validation:</u>** Documented evidence that a process(e.g. sterilization) does what it purports to do.

Organization and Personnel

- Deals with responsibilities of quality control unit, employees and consultants

- All personnel engaged in manufacture, processing, packing or holding of drug product

- Including those in supervisory positions, are required to have education, training and/or experience needed to fulfill the assigned responsibility.

Buildings and facilities

- Include design, structural features and functional aspects of buildings and facilities

- Each building structure, space, design and placement of equipment must be such to enable thorough cleaning, inspection and safe and effective use for designated operations

- Proper consideration given to factors--- water quality standards, security, materials used for floors, walls and ceilings, lighting etc..

- Segregated quarantine areas for raw materials and product components subject to quality control approval.

- holding areas, storage areas, weighing rooms, sterile areas, control of heat, humidity, temp. and ventilation

- work in manufacture, processing, packing or holding of pharmaceutical product must be logged in, inspected and signed off

Equipment

- Each piece must be of appropriate design and size

- Suitably located to facilitate operations for use, cleaning and maintenance

- Equipments surfaces and parts must not interact with processes or product's components so as to alter purity, strength or quality.

- SOP must be followed for use, maintenance, and cleaning

- Logs and records MUST be kept

- Automated equipment and computers must be calibrated routinely and validated for accuracy

- Filters used in injectable products should not release fibers.

Production and Process Controls

- Written procedures required

- Deviation from written procedures must be recorded and justified.

- In case of automated control operations, equipments validated regularly for precision.

- All equipment, containers must be labelled

- Records maintained

Packaging and labeling control

- Labeling for each variation in drug product – strength, dosage form or quantity of contents- must be stored separately with suitable identification

- Obsolete and outdated labels must be destroyed

- Access to storage area must be limited to authorized personnel.

- All materials must be withheld until approved and released by quality control unit

- Before labelling operations commence, labelling facilities must be inspected to ensure

that all drug products and labels have been removed from previous operations

- labels meet legal requirements for content

Carry-expiration dating and lot no.

Holding and Distribution

- Finished pharmaceuticals must be quarantined in storage until released by quality control unit.

- Products must be stored and shipped under conditions that do not affect product quality.

- Oldest approved stock is distributed first.

Records and Reports

- Production, control and distribution records must be maintained for at least a year following expiration date of a product batch Records must include:

1.Name and strength of product

2.Dosage Form

3.Quantitative amounts of components and dosage units

4. Complete manufacturing and control procedures

5. Specifications

6. In-process controls

7. Calibration of instruments

8. Distribution records

9. Dated and employee identified records

- These records must document that each step in production, control, packaging, labeling and distribution of product was accomplished and approved by quality control unit.

- Operator's and supervisor's signatures, initials or written or electronic identification codes are required.

- All records must be made available at the time of inspection by FDA officials

Learning outcomes

- Definition

- Main Components

- Principles of GMP

- Standards for CGMP

CHAPTER 10

Good Compounding Practices (GCP)

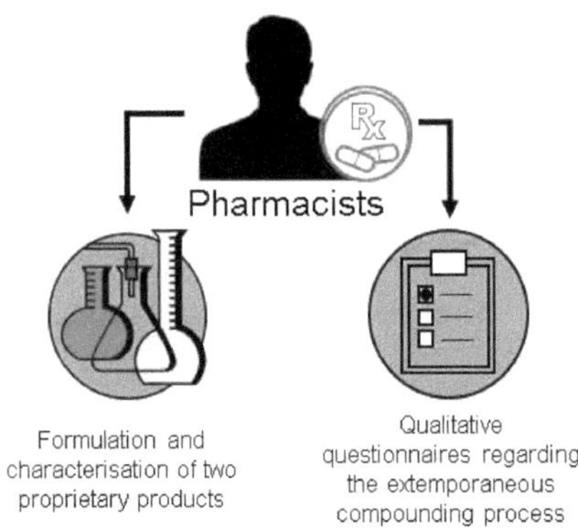

Objectives

➥ General Principles

➥ Characteristics of Compounding

➥ General Steps in the Compounding Process

➥ Problems that often occur in Compounding

➡ Current Good Compounding Practices

GENERAL PRINCIPLES

➡ Compounding is an integral part of pharmacy practice and is essential to the provision of health care

➡ **Compounding :**

    ➡ The act of combining two or more ingredients in the preparation of prescription.

    ➡ The ingredients intended for use in the compounding of a drug product.

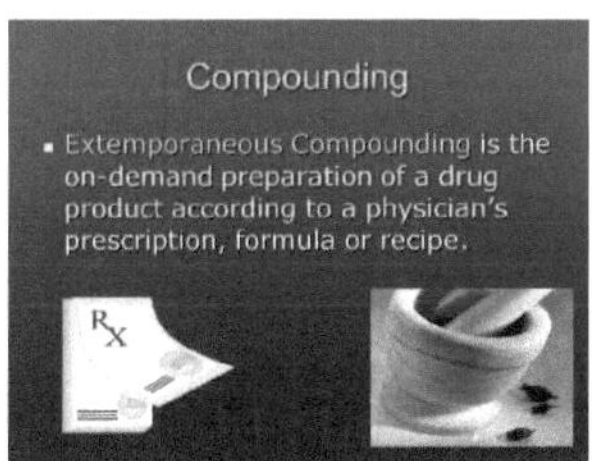

Compounding is defined as:

➡ "to combine, mix of substances or alteration of dosage form or strength or delivery system of a medicinal product tailored to the needs and quantity of an individual; includes the combination of two or more compounded preparation or substances."

A compounded preparation should be prepared only in circumstances when:

➡ a) A registered product is unavailable in the market.

- b) A registered product with similar therapeutic effect is unavailable in the market.

- c) A registered product is unsuitable (e.g. if a patient experiencing allergy to an excipient in the registered product).

- d) When undertaking research sanctioned by a recognised human research ethics committee.

- e) A treatment requires tailored dosage strengths/forms for patients with unique needs (for example, an infant).

Compounding may include the following:

- Preparation of drug dosage forms for both human and animal patients

- Preparation of drugs or devices in anticipation of prescription drug orders, on the basis of routine, regularly observed prescribing patterns.

- Reconstitution or manipulation of commercial products that may require the addition of one or more ingredients.

- Preparation of drugs or devices for the purposes of, or as an incident to, research (clinical or academic), teaching, or chemical analysis, and

- Preparation of drugs and devices for prescriber's office use where permitted by federal and state law.

RESPONSIBLE PERSON

- Compounding preparation shall be done by a Responsible Person as stated below:

- a) a pharmacist or a person working under the immediate personal supervision of a pharmacist.

- b) a person acting in the course of his duties who is employed in hospital or dispensary.

- c) a fully registered medical practitioner or a dental practitioner or a veterinary practitioner or a person working under the immediate personal

- supervision of such a practitioner if the drug in question is for the use of such practitioner or of his patient.

- Note: For poison compounding, it should be done in accordance with section 12 of the Poisons Act 1952.

Characteristics of Compounding

- To properly perform compounding, a pharmacist must consider several aspects, namely:

1. Administrative Aspect

- The administrative aspect relates to prescriptions.

In here, pharmacists check on the administrative completeness of the prescription, particularly:

- Date,

- Information,

- International Statistical Classification of Diseases and Related Health Problems,

- Doctor's Name and Signature,

- Inscription,

- Subscription, and Directions for Use.

2. Pharmaceutical Aspect

➡ The pharmaceutical aspect covers safety, effectiveness, and stability of the drug and acceptance of the drug by the patient.

3. Clinical Aspect

➡ The clinical aspect encompasses drug indications, effectiveness, safety, and compatibility of dosage forms, and review of patient compliance.

General Steps in the Compounding Process

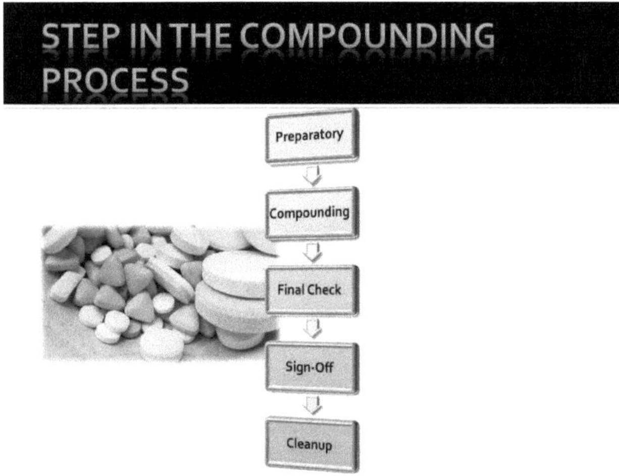

<u>**Preparation phase:**</u>

- ➡ 1. Receiving and checking for completeness and authenticity of the recipe.

- ➡ 2. Clarifying with the doctor or patient about any missing information.

- ➡ 3. Calculating drug dosages and checking for drug interactions.

- ➡ 4. Calculating the amount of drugs and excipients to be used.

- ➡ 5. Maintaining proper hygiene and the cleanliness of the compounding area.

<u>**Compounding phase:**</u>

- ➡ 6. Dispensing all the necessary ingredients.

- ➡ 7. Careful review of the ingredients.

- ➡ 8. Compounding based on the appropriate technique.

<u>**Final Phase:**</u>

- 9. Checking for indication, weight variation, and homogeneity of formulation made.

- 10. Logging of information in compounding books.

- 11. Labeling of the prepared drug.

- 12. Cleaning of both compounding and storage areas.

- 13. Giving (dispensing) medication to patient.

Problems that often occur in compounding

- When compounding, pharmacists often encounter several problems, which can be categorized into five:

1. Quality Problems

- These involve the temperature and humidity of the room influencing the stability of the drug, the readiness of pharmacy personnel in conducting compounding, particularly the wearing of personal protective equipment as in laboratory coats, masks, and gloves.

- In addition, the cleanliness of equipment used and the presence of contamination are other factors that cause problems in compounding.

2. Calculation Problems

- These involve problems related to the computation of suitable doses, amount of drugs and excipients to be weighed, and appropriate dilution.

3. Dosage Form Problems

- These problems are encountered with drugs having varying dosage strengths within the dosage form. For example, a drug in the form of coated tablet, such as delayed-release or sustained-release, cannot be crushed to obtain a smaller dose as doing so will damage the existing matrix system.

4. Stability Problems

- These problems encompass those which are related to

    - drug storage,

    - drug packaging, and

    - special treatments/mixing techniques.

    - An example is the mixing of menthol and camphor, which can cause a decrease in melting point (eutectic point).

5. Incompatibility Problems

- These are problems of serious consideration by pharmacists, which may fall under the following categories:

- **physical incompatibility**: an example of which is color change

- **chemical incompatibility**: as seen in drug degradation

- **pharmacological incompatibility**: which is an incompatibility that results to toxicity

Storage

- Compounding chemicals should be stored in tightly closed, light-resistant containers at room temperature; some chemicals, however, require refrigeration.

- Chemicals should be stored off the floor, preferably on shelves in a clean, dry environment.

- Commercial drugs to be used in the compounding process should be removed from cartons and boxes before they are stored in the compounding area.

- The temperatures of the storage areas, including refrigerators and freezers, should be monitored and recorded at least weekly.

- Labelling: Labelling should be done according to state and federal regulations.

Usually, labelling information includes the :

- (1) generic or chemical names of the active ingredients,

- (2) strength or quantity,

- (3) pharmacy lot number,

- (4) beyond-use date,

- (5) any special storage requirements.

Current Good Compounding Practices

- ➡ In recent years pharmacists have increased the practice of compounding patient-specific medications

Reasons

- 1. Many patients need drug dosages or strengths that are not commercially available.

- 2. Many patients need dosage forms such as suppositories, oral liquids, or topical that are not commercially available

- 3. Many patients are allergic to excipients in commercially available products

- 4. Children's medications must be prepared as liquids, flavored to enhance compliance and prepared as lozenges, gum drops and lollipops

- 5. Some medications are not very stable, require preparation, dispensing every few days

- 6. Many products reported in literature, but not manufactured yet, so pharmacists can compound them for patient and physicians use.

- 7. Many physicians desire products in innovative ways, pharmacist work to solve medication problems.

As extent of compounding increased, many standard setting agencies and regulatory bodies came to ensure quality compounded products

In mid 1990's activities to establish guidelines for pharmaceutical compounding.

U.S. Pharmacopeia-National Formulary

- Chapter on "Pharmacy Compounding Practices" was published and became official in 1996.

➡ First compounding monographs became official in 1998.

CHAPTER talks about

➡ A) Compounding environment

➡ B) Stability

➡ C) Ingredient selection and calculations

➡ D) Checklist for acceptable strength, quality and purity

➡ E) Compounded preparations

➡ F) Compounding Process

➡ G) Compounding records and documents

➡ H) Quality control

➡ i) Patient counseling

➡ Introduction discusses difference between compounding and manufacturing.

➡ Compounding differs from manufacturing in specific-practitioner-patient-pharmacist relationship, quantity of medication prepared in anticipation of receiving a prescription and conditions of sale which are limited to specific prescription orders.

➡ The National Association of Boards of Pharmacy promulgated the Good Compounding Practices.

➡ Adopted, modified and adopted by many states.

➡ Chapters, monographs for USP-NF.

- Resulted in section of Food and Drug Administration Modernization Act of 1997

- This was to support pharmacists right to compound, with some guidelines.

Food and Drug Modernization Act, 1997

- Purpose was to ensure patients' access to individualized drug therapy and prevent unnecessary FDA regulation of health professional practice

- Act exempted pharmacy compounding from several regulatory requirements but did not exempt drug manufacturing.

- Act states that a compounded product is exempt if drug product is compounded for

- an individual patient based on unsolicited receipt of valid prescription order approved by prescribing practitioner that compounded product is necessary for identified patient.

- Act removed any doubt that compounding is legal under FDC Act

- Congress has clearly recognized the importance of compounding.

<u>National Association of Boards of Pharmacy</u>

- GCP applicable to state licensed Pharmacies developed by Board discusses 8 recommendations

- **<u>Sub part A</u>** General Provisions provides 2 imp. Definitions of compounding and manufacturing

- **<u>Sub part B</u>**, Organization and personnel discusses responsibilities of pharmacists

- and other personnel engaged in compounding.

- also stresses that only personnel authorized by responsible pharmacist shall be in immediate vicinity of drug compounding operation.

- **<u>Subpart C</u>**: Drug Compounding facilities describes area that should be set aside for compounding, either sterile or not.

- Special attention required for radiopharmaceuticals and for products requiring precautions to minimize contamination e.g. penicillin.

- **<u>Subpart D</u>:** Equipments--- appropriate design, adequate size, suitably located to facilitate operation for its intended use, cleaning and maintenance

- **<u>Subpart E</u>:** Control of components and drug product containers, closures, describes packaging requirements for compounded products

- **<u>Subpart F</u>:** Drug compounding controls discusses written procedures to ensure that finished products are of proper identity, strength, quality and purity as labeled.

- **<u>Subpart G</u>:**labeling control of excess products and records and reports, describes records that are required under these guidelines.

- All pharmacists should become familiar with the individual state requirements

Learning Outcomes

- General Principles, Characteristics of Compounding, General Steps in the Compounding Process, Problems that often occur in Compounding, Current Good Compounding Practices

References

Textbooks / Other Learning Resources

1. A textbook of pharmaceutical analysis, 3rd Ed. By Kenneth a. Connors, Wiley-Interscience, 605 Third Avenue, New York, NY 10016. (Latest edition)

2. Pharmaceutical Analysis. A text book for Pharmacy Students and Pharmaceutical Chemists, 3rd Ed, David G Watson, Churchill Livingstone, UK, (Latest edition)

3. British Pharmacopoeia

4. L. Lachman, Theory and Practice of Industrial Pharmacy Lea & Febiger; 3rd edition,(1986) (Latest edition)

5. Cartersen J.T and Rodes C.T Drug Stability. Principles and Practices (3rd Edition Marcel,Dekker, New York 2000)

6. Allen, LV, Nicholas G, Ansel HC. Ansel's Pharmaceutical Dosage Forms and Drug Delivery Systems, Lippincott Williams & Wilkins, 2011. (Latest edition)

7. Aulton, M.E. Pharmaceutics. The Science of dosage form design, (2nd ed.), Churchill Livingstone, 2001.

8. Meyer R. Rosen, Harry's Cosmeticology, Chemical publishing company, USA. (Latest Edition)

9. Pharmaceutical Technology. A Practical Manual, Sushma Talegaonkar, Pharma Med Press/BSP Books, 2018.

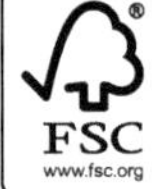

Printed by Books on Demand GmbH, Norderstedt / Germany